For V

It's well i my soul

Bud Miller

October '04

LIKE HIS TEACHER

Memoirs of a
Rural Kansas Physician

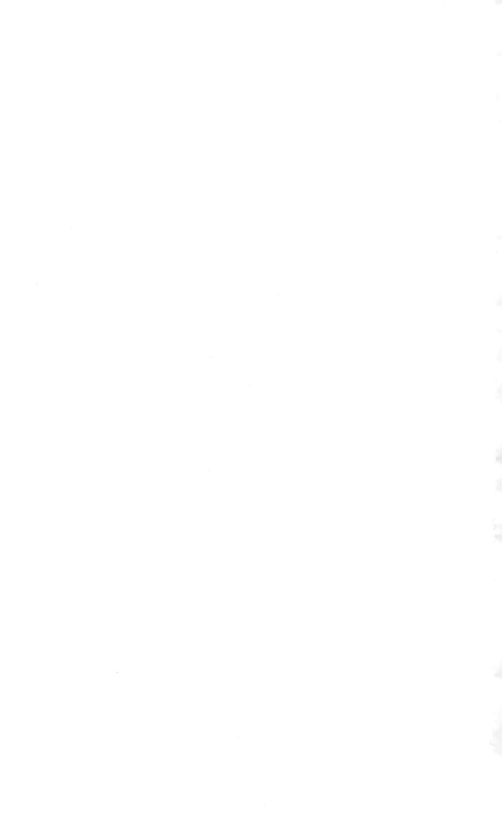

LIKE HIS TEACHER

Memoirs of a Rural Kansas Physician

By

DR. BUD GOLLIER

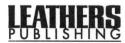

A division of Squire Publishers, Inc.
4500 College Blvd.
Leawood, KS 66211
1/888/888-7696

Copyright 2002
Printed in the United States

ISBN: 1-58597-145-6 (Hard back)
ISBN: 1-58597-157-X (Soft cover)

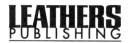

A division of Squire Publishers, Inc.
4500 College Blvd.
Leawood, KS 66211
1/888/888-7696

This book is dedicated to
Big Nelle and Robert C. Cooper

This is a memoir, but please understand that (to any writer with a good imagination) all memoirs are false. A fiction writer's memory is an especially imperfect provider of detail; we can always imagine a better detail than the one we can remember. The correct detail is rarely, exactly, what happened; the most truthful detail is what could have happened ... or what should have. Being a writer is a strenuous marriage between careful observation and just as carefully imagining the truths you haven't had the opportunity to see.

— John Irving
Trying to Save Piggy Sneed

The Struggle

Fragile lady,
You lie so still.
Your eyes don't see.
Your ears don't hear.
You move not with purpose.
Your chest moves
When the air enters your lungs,
But the air does nothing.
For the cancer, like a parasite,
Steals the oxygen from the air
And robs you, the host,
Of oxygen,
Of nutrients,
Of calories,
Of life itself.

The cancer demands its own survival
At your expense,
The gnawing pain the only
Reminder of its presence,
Felt only by you, fragile lady.
Yet you do not move
Or speak out.
But we sense you do hear,
And see,
And feel.
Only your response is numbed.
You know we are here.
You know we care.
We leave the room,
Your family and I,
To talk of things you need not hear.
We talk of care and comfort.
We leave the struggle to you
And your uninvited guest.
We pray for release
And Quietness.

ACKNOWLEDGMENTS

Over a fifteen-year period of time there are many people who have given support to or, rather, tolerated my writing project. First of all in this effort, as in the rest of my life, my wife, Mary Lynn, has been by my side only occasionally asking where I want this pile of papers to go. Of my transcriptionists, Jane Harris deserves hazardous duty pay as she was there at the first with the handwritten sheaves of paper. The work has had at least eight different titles and has moved from yellow legal pads to dictated additions and finally to the word processor where one misplaced keypunch could lose the entire project. Loda Newcomb, Debbie Barkley, Teresa Powers, Dianne Caryl and finally Frances Wells helped put together much of the transcription.

For the history of Ottawa and Ottawa University, I am indebted to John Mark Lambertson. For spiritual counsel, The Reverends Henry Roberts, Roger Fredrikson, James McCrossen and Steven Van Ostran guided me at times. John Peterson helped guide my awkward literary style by encouraging me to read great books to understand how to tell a story. A creative writing class taught by Lora Reiter and Dexter Westrum at Ottawa University helped direct me.

Finally my family read and edited the nearly finished story. There is always something to change. It is far from perfect. However, the flaws, though not intentional, remind the author that he, like everyone else, is a work in progress.

BOOK I

The Way It Was

ONE

The primary care doctor of 60 years ago was free of the specter of retrospective review and free to care for patients based on need and trust.

HE HAD BEEN A COUNTRY DOCTOR for 35 years and had seen his calling evolve from country doctor to general practitioner to family physician. He liked general practitioner best. "Just a G.P.," he would say proudly when asked his specialty. "I take care of people."

When he died, his wife asked me if I would like to review his personal papers. "He kept a lot of old books," she told me. I jumped at the chance. He had saved his medical textbooks, journals, appointment books and daily ledgers from 1939 through 1958.

I began with July 1939. His wife had told me that was his first full month. The entries were recorded in the doctor's careful hand. Of course, he couldn't afford a receptionist or secretary. The charges were in his hand as well, so he was the bookkeeper, too. I sensed he also served as nurse in the early days. The first page listed 12 patients. In the column headed services rendered, he entered his documentation, usually a short, one-word description. No need to be expansive with medical records in 1939. The usual entry was "call" with a charge of $1. An "early A.M." call at home was $2, or a call "with med" or "with exam" was $2. The next column was labeled "cash" and was usually filled with the same figure listed in the charge column.

The list went on: Night Call — $4; House Call with spinal puncture — $10; Delivery (home) — $35; Delivery (home with episiotomy) — $45; tonsillectomy (home) — $30 ($5 to Dr. Barr — anesthesia). What a treasure I had!

The next entry threw me — Mrs. J.E. Decker, Williamsburg, blood transfusion (home) — $10. The next day he listed Mrs. Decker again, re-check — no charge. It had been a Sunday. He had driven 16 miles on a Sunday to re-check the patient, and he wasn't even worried about a malpractice claim.

Another entry listed Mrs. Evert — home delivery (episiotomy) — $45. The next three days he listed Mrs. Evert with infant — no charge.

There were frequent notations for med. — 25 cents. And then Mrs. Jones — med, (cab) — 35 cents. I could picture the doctor looking out his office window, waiting for the cab, then walking out to hand the cabby the package and a dime. He also mailed medicine for 60 cents. It must have been cheaper to send it by cab. Maybe that hasn't changed. His records showed no mention of a diagnosis or type of medication. He was just meeting what he perceived as a need.

I was amazed at the breadth of his medical experience: R.M. Clogston; fracture (tibia) cast $6; Kit Harbison appendectomy — $110; Larry Barnett, pack nose — $1; Mrs. Lowrance lance boil — $2; Mrs. F.H. Carr (four kids) (50 cents each) — $2. The next notation said bellboy — North American Hotel call (med) — $1. Perhaps he gave the employee a discount, then a country call for $4.

I read through the rest of the month and was stopped in my tracks with two entries, both Saturday night calls. One was Ann Hutchins, Room 220, North American Hotel; the other was Mr. Armstrong, Room 8, Nelson Hotel. Both charges were $3. I imagined a phone call on a Saturday night from the local Hallmark Inn requesting a doctor's visit. I wouldn't know whether to call the police, sheriff or National Guard to accompany me.

Then a six-month miscarriage (home)— $35 and a follow-up the next day — no charge. And an emergency call, X-ray, set arm — $35 (with cast). Next, Milo Hewitt suture — $5 paid; Mr. and Mrs. Spears call Homewood (two) — $5; Mrs. Herb Sheldon suture thumb — $3; Charles Mahoney tonsillectomy — $25, Leon Mahoney tonsillectomy — $25, Bennett boys four shots — $3.

There were several entries for intramuscular liver extract $1, a traditional remedy for anemia. He had two patients receiving shots of Thio-bismol twice a week at $1 per shot, following a spinal puncture at home. There was no mention of a laboratory report for syphilis, but I remembered bismuth was an early treatment for syphilis. One of those patients is under my care in a nursing home at this time. I had an answer for his murmur of aortic insufficiency.

At the end of the month, he listed expenses:

Nurse	$90.00
Office	55.00
Laundry	3.25
Telephone	11.89
Drugs & Supplies	55.42
Stamps	4.20
Chamber of Commerce	3.00
Welfare Board	2.50
Total Expenses	($225.26)

Then came the monthly balance:

Total charges	$160.25
Total cash received	148.25
Total expenses	225.26
Net profit (or loss)	($ 77.01)

Not exactly a booming start, but he was collecting over 90 cents on the dollar. That was before HMO and government reimbursement policies had taken their toll, I thought, as I reflected on my current collection percentage of 70 percent. I quickly glanced through the next few months. His income was steady. The expenses seemed reasonable. Something was missing. It hit me suddenly – he had no insurance expense. Surely he had liability insurance. I turned to August, then September and October. I noted by the end of September his summary showed:

Year-to-Date	Cash	$882.00
	Expenses	(698.00)
Profit (or loss)		$184.00

Finally, he was in the black. Then in November 1939, there was a new entry: Medical Liability Insurance — $7.50. I raced through the next few months. Was his premium monthly or quarterly? The next entry was February for $4. Then in October, again $4. So his malpractice insurance was $8 per year. He would have it paid after seeing four patients. I quickly calculated that I would have to see 400 patients to cover my most recent premium. I settled down in a comfortable chair and read the ledgers through 1958. It was good reading. I sensed a man who loved his work and his patients. People trusted and admired this man as much as he admired them.

It was a cash-and-carry business — all one-on-one. He was often paid by trade. One patient regularly brought eggs. An office call was paid by "chicken" on more than one occasion.

No third party, no lawyers. Just a man serving his friends. No concern for malpractice, collections, third-party review or assault by drug addicts or criminals.

I sensed his involvement with his patients as he shared grief with the Rice family in 1941. His style was to make short entries, and the entry noting the Rice family car wreck was uncharacteristically detailed. He described Mr. Rice's fractured clavicle and maxilla, and eyelid laceration. He described Mrs. Rice's lacerated arm and broken leg, including a one-hour surgery to control bleeding and repair torn muscles in her arm. There were no charges noted for either. There were two blank spaces and then two haunting entries: Rice boy — died; Rice girl — died. I could feel the tension and sense the drama in that 1941 rural hospital emergency room. I understood why there had been no charge.

I sensed the fulfillment that fueled his dedication. I sensed his love for his profession. He had been my physician when I was a boy and he had inspired me to follow in his footsteps. I was now reading a part of the story I had not known.

I finally read the entry of my birth, which was assisted by a Kansas City obstetrician. I read quickly through the late 1940s and 1950s. Then an entry caught my eye. It was July 1951. Mrs. White, N. Cherry — delivery (home) — $50 ($10 to pilot). I called the physician's wife. She remembered it well.

"There were no doctors on the north side of the river. The police called and said they had received a radio call for help. A lady was in labor. Old Mary (the Marais des Cygne River) was out and he couldn't get across. He went out to the airport and found a pilot to fly him over the flood. They landed in a pasture over there someplace. After the delivery, he had them radio that he would come home when the flood was over. He didn't like to fly."

As I read his journal, I sensed his call to provide service was based on need. I remembered a warning he gave me during my youth when I told him I wanted to be a doctor. Congress had passed legislation signed by President Johnson. It was to be called Medicare. He warned it would be a disaster. "It will place a devastating burden on the budget. It will be good for doctors, for a while. I don't charge my elderly patients if they can't pay. Politicians don't understand that. Now I'll be able to charge for everyone I see. Many elderly people can afford care, but they'll let the government foot the bill. When they realize how expensive it is, the government will begin accusing the doctor for overcharging and seeing people who don't need to see a doctor. Then the bureaucrats will control the fees and pay what suits them. Finally, they will tell the doctor what to do, and if he doesn't cooperate, the patients will have to see one who will play ball with the government. Patients will lose their freedom of choice, and there will be bureaucrats to run the program and we will have to pay them, too. Americans like to have their freedom. They'll raise hell when they lose their freedom to choose their doctor, but it will be too late. I'd advise you to hold out as long as you can, because in the final analysis, the politicians will choose to blame the doctors for the high cost."

I reflected on the current health care environment. We still teach our doctors to provide care based on need. The cost of service does not figure into the equation in traditional medical education. But doctors now must learn to adapt on their own. Doctors are dreamers. They hope for the best in their patients and apply that optimism to their prayers for their profession.

But the fate of medical care is in the hands of politicians.

No one is going to speak for the doctors or the patients. Health care is a major expense that will be controlled by those who set our national priorities. It was a good time 60 years ago, but those days are gone. The doctor sensed it would come to this. The reviewing bureaucrats are cloaked as peers as they mix with the flock, but a wolf is not hard to spot. They will mean the end of quality medicine based on need. It will come to cost effectiveness.

No longer is it enough to do the best one can. Patients have come to expect perfection. These great expectations, with flames fanned by the winds generated in the legal profession, have found a virtual tinderbox in today's litigious society. The doctor and patient have become adversaries. The human bond that drew them together is stretched to the limit. Doctors may be able to overcome the strain, but it takes added time to build the trust that strengthens the bond. Time is hard to find. It is a high price for a special profession, but it is worth the price.

The spirit of the doctor still lives, but physicians must adapt to changing times and patients must be realistic in their expectations or the doctor's essence will only be a memory.

The doctor was my father. How right he was.

TWO

IT HAD BEEN A MAD-HOUSE at the office. I got home about 5:30 p.m. and took a quick glance at the newspaper while Mary Lynn was getting dinner ready. The kids were all enjoying the early spring weather and were all involved in different outdoor activities. John was shooting baskets across the street and Bo was at golf practice. Sara Jane was babysitting.

The dinner schedule was going to be hectic once again as we had to be at the forum at 7 o'clock. As Mary Lynn put the dinner on the table, Bo, John and Sara Jane rushed in together. I led the prayer and we all began chatting at once about the day's activities.

"How did the golf go today, Bo?"

"Okay, Dad."

"How were you hitting the ball?"

"Okay."

"How were you putting?"

"Okay."

I took a deep breath and paused before trying to find the question that would break through the teen-age shield of indifference.

"What are you going to tell them tonight, Dad?"

I was taken aback by Bo's question.

"I'm not certain, Bo, but it will be mostly about what this town has meant to me and how much I want it always to stay a special place."

"You'll do great," he grinned at me, his obligatory inquiry behind him.

"I'm going over to Barry's to shoot baskets."

I got up and walked out onto the front lawn. The grass needed cutting. The dandelions were beginning to erupt. It always amazed me that such a beautiful yellow bloom as a dandelion was classified as a weed and not a flower. I then remembered how they would look in a few weeks scattering their seeds with the wind throughout the neighborhood. It also occurred to me that scientists had predicted that cockroaches would be the only survivors of World War III. The cockroaches will have dandelions to admire. I remembered I would have to call the lawn care service and tell them their sure-fire dandelion killer hadn't worked.

I waved at Bob Soph and Merle Price visiting in the alley across the street. I sat down on the front porch. A feeling of well-being washed over me. I felt good. My son was again taking it for granted that I wouldn't embarrass him, and I knew what I was going to say at the Chamber of Commerce "Meet the Candidates" forum.

I knew why I had always dreamed of raising a family in Ottawa, Kansas. I knew why it fit the criteria as a setting for helping my children learn how to relate to people and to respect others' rights and understand their needs and what they feel. Dad had always said that I should not judge another man until I had walked in his shoes a few miles.

In Ottawa, we all sensed each other's basic needs and shared in each other's children's successes and failures. I could remember the concern displayed by my parents when Don Harrison, four years ahead of me in school, lost his leg to bone cancer while in high school and the thrill the community felt when he bounced back to continue his education and become the anchorman on the WIBW-TV evening news in Topeka, on his way to CNN in Atlanta.

I could remember how my father had worried about Kent Granger, the son of a good friend and one of Ottawa High School's most popular students, when Kent was in an iron lung with polio. My father was thrilled for Kent when he left the hospital and battled his way through college and Stanford Law School on his way to becoming one of Kansas City's most successful attorneys.

We all felt a part of each triumph because we had all been intimately involved in the trials and battles leading to the achievement. We cherished the victory as if it had been won by one of our own family members.

The high school auditorium was packed. I sat on the stage with seven other candidates. I'm sure we all looked nervous and apprehensive, but I was not nervous at all. Strangely, I was loving every minute of it. I had paid my dues. My nervous moments had been during my rehabilitation when I questioned whether I had any future at all, whether I could enjoy life and be an effective husband and father. I knew that while I wanted to win the election, it was more important to me that I had the self-confidence to be on stage and be considered a candidate.

I saw Connie Thompson on the back row. She and her husband, Jerry, had been in my high school class. Jerry was a successful contractor and was on the stage as a candidate for city commission.

As I looked around the audience, I noted that the room was filled with neighbors, friends, patients and many people I had known all my life.

The moderator got my attention when he said, "The next candidate for the school board is Dr. Bud Gollier." The lump in my throat disappeared as I took a deep breath and adjusted the microphone.

"Twenty-seven years ago there was a Chamber of Commerce banquet at Eugene Field Elementary School. The theme of the evening was 'Bring Industry to Ottawa.' Reverend Roger Fredrikson of the First Baptist Church moderated a panel discussion after dinner. The first speaker was J.R. 'Duke' Cheney, who spoke of transportation. He mentioned that Ottawa was served by two railroads, the Santa Fe and the Missouri Pacific, and that two highways passed through town. He spoke of plans to build an interstate highway network that was to be known as I-35 that would link Ottawa with Kansas City, 50 miles to the northeast and connect with the Kansas Turnpike at Emporia, 55 miles southwest.

"The second speaker was Lamar Phillips, who spoke of his work with the U.S. Army Corps of Engineers and plans to control the ravaging floods of the Marais des Cygnes River by building reservoirs upstream to impound the water and meet recreational needs in the summer. There would also be an elaborate system of dikes and levees complete with a moveable gate at the river bridge to keep flood water out of downtown Ottawa.

"The third speaker was Milo Hewitt, the inspiration of the Ottawa Industrial Development Committee of the Chamber of Commerce. Milo spoke of plans for an Industrial Park on the outskirts of town, complete with attractive financing to attract new industry to Ottawa.

"I was the last speaker that evening, a 17-year-old high school senior, the president of the student council, who had been pirated out of his high school basketball practice by Rev. Fredrikson with the promise of a belly-full of Colonel Sanders' Kentucky Fried Chicken in exchange for a brief discussion on the subject, 'Why Ottawa is a good town to grow up in.' I remember running home to change clothes with a thousand thoughts and memories racing through my mind. I knew the knots in my stomach were going to take care of my appetite. What could I possibly say to the community leaders? I made some quick notes so I wouldn't panic and make a fool of myself.

"On that evening, I told the Chamber of Commerce that Ottawa was a good town to grow up in because of its friendly people, its many recreational opportunities, its proximity to Kansas City and the University of Kansas, only 25 miles north, its community spirit and its rich and colorful heritage. Ottawa was founded in 1837 by the Reverend and Mrs. Jotham Meeker as a Baptist mission for the Ottawa Indians. The couple laid the foundation for future White-Indian cooperation. The principal founders of the city in 1864 included Isaac S. Kalloch, a Baptist minister from the East; C.C. Hutchinson, a government agent to the Ottawa Indians, and John Tecumseh 'Tauy' Jones, an adopted chief and spiritual leader of the Ottawas. These same men, led by Tauy Jones, established Ottawa University in 1865, which today is a four-year liberal arts college which serves as testimony to the community's dedication to education.

"Ottawa has survived floods, drought and depression. With a population stable at 11,000 and agriculture as its primary economic base, the people have learned to deal with many uncertainties. Most of all, I said that night, Ottawa is a good town to grow up in because of its excellent schools. The schools embody the educational commitment of our founding fathers.

"I have now come full circle. I have returned to raise my children in the community that holds a warm spot in my heart. I now see my children enrolled in those same schools that are responsible for whatever success I have enjoyed. However, I see a school system that is falling short in the ideals that have given us strength. I see a dropout rate above the state average. I see a failure to motivate children to enroll in higher level courses — a physics course was not filled at Ottawa High School last year. Our athletic teams have fallen on hard times. We no longer encourage children to push themselves. We must pursue excellence. Our children are our greatest resources. They are like diamonds in the rough. We have the obligation to polish them, help them reach their full potential and help them feel good about themselves. I share the dreams of our founding fathers, of 'Duke' Cheney, of Lamar Phillips, of Milo Hewitt and of Roger Fredrikson. That is why I am running for the school board. It is nice to be back."

Many of those at this forum reminded me, with misty eyes, that they had been there 27 years ago. They had forgotten how far we had come with I-35 and the flood control project in place as if they had always been there. I reminded them that we have a long way to go. Twenty-seven years before my father had been on the school board while I was in high school. The more things change, the more things stay the same.

It is hard for me to believe that six years previously I was expected to die. The question was survival. The prospects for purposeful and functional recovery were grim, but my wife, Mary Lynn, my family and friends did not give up on me and I could not let them down.

I am told I was in a coma for more than two weeks. The doctors were gathered outside the Intensive Care Unit when my father-in-law came by to visit. He overheard one of them say, "I don't think he is going to make it." Another one chimed in and said, "Have you told his wife?" The first doctor replied, "She would never believe me. She told me this morning she thought he tried to open his eyes."

I cannot make any sense out of it. It all seems like a bad dream now. I can vividly remember fleeting parts of my hospitalization, but most of it is a blur. I remember walking across the street to the hospital with my father and telling the hospital volunteer I would walk to my room and then losing that battle as my father insisted I use the wheelchair. Most of all, I remember the pounding headache and the sense of relief that I was finally going to have the problem solved. The high blood pressure worried me, but I knew the doctors would get it down right away. After all, I had dealt with acute hypertensive crises in my patients and I knew it was just a matter of starting an IV, giving medication and observing the response to see which medicine would be most effective. I remember talk of a spinal tap and a CAT scan. I then remember standing up and saying to Mary Lynn, "I can't stand it!"

It was then that I had a seizure as a result of a brain hemorrhage. The extent of the hemorrhage is the factor that determines survival and functional impairment. Rapid treatment of the seizure and lowering of the blood pressure are the critical measures to limit the extent of the damage.

This is the story of an illness and an uncommon recovery. It is a story of survival through a medical emergency that was dependent on family support and prayer. Steps in the recovery were vivid, but putting the story together has been perplexing. Mary Lynn and my brother, Fred, told me the nurses did not pay much attention to me the first few days I was in the hospital. My room was down at the end of the hall specifically where it was quiet and no one would bother me since it was assumed I was suffering from stress and needed complete relaxation. My dad just shook his head and did not want to talk about it. My mother said that sort of thing happens everywhere. "Just be glad you are alive," was her usual reply. I was more an object than a participant in the recovery. The direction of my journey through life has given me a great opportunity to reflect on the meaningful experiences of my early years. These experiences, by themselves, are isolated and only in review after a crisis do the parts come together and have a sensible relationship to one another. The ability to deal comfortably with conflict is a result of understanding oneself and learning to ride easily in the harness, as Robert Frost wrote.

To understand oneself, it is important to have a view of the sum total of personal development. An understanding of the important ingredients of the social being is essential to an effective resolution of conflict.

Faith, trust, responsibility, respect, commitment and consistency are all integral parts of a developing personality. In order to relate to others meaningfully, it is critical for one to be firmly in control of his moral position. If there is confusion in one's values, he will relate to another in an unpredictable fashion. The net effect will be as if two ships are passing at night in a storm without instruments to give a sense of position. They will have to rely on luck to avoid a catastrophic collision.

The fabric in my life has been provided by strong parents, religious instruction that was allowed to develop independently, the good fortune to marry a woman who is my perfect complement and an implied expectation that I was going to succeed.

This is a story of family support as well as prayer support. The family and community support helped kindle a determination that culminated in self-preservation that would not be denied. It is the story of a journey from death's door to complete recovery, thanks to the tireless support of a loving wife and family who never quit encouraging me and never lost faith in my recovery.

The underlying thread in the story is that faith in God, along with family support and encouragement, can lead to an unexpected happy conclusion in the most discouraging cases. I hope the reader will learn that we are not at the mercy of the system and that we do have control over our destiny if we are committed to surviving and have goals for the future and a purpose in life. We must all take control of our lives as we are ultimately responsible for what happens to us. I hope this realization will help others survive crises in their lives.

This story also points out some potential flaws in the

medical care delivery system. I must share some responsibility for that, but I hope my experience will have a positive effect on our profession. Let me tell you my story.

Mary Lynn says the story began when I had a bad fall while skiing in Breckenridge, Colorado. Mother says it began when I met Mary Lynn. Dad says it began when he rushed me to Metropolitan Hospital with a pounding headache. But I think it all began in the middle of a July night on the muddy banks of Wea Creek in Miami County in eastern Kansas. It was 1945. I was five years old, cold and soaking wet. Dad and my grandfather were trying to turn the boat back over and Dad was saying, "Nelle isn't going to like this one bit!"

That was the night I first realized the importance of meaningful family relationships. I did not know that the strength of that relationship would give me the strength to survive another near disaster 33 years later.

THREE

MY MOTHER WAS RAISED in a small town in central Missouri. Her childhood centered around church and family. She tells of family get-togethers nearly every weekend. Her father had three brothers and two sisters who lived near the small town of Marshall, Missouri, the county seat of Saline county. Her mother had a brother who also lived in the community. There were 11 cousins, all nearly the same age, who were very close during their youth. Family tradition was to give children two names, so mother was christened Nelle Marshall Barnhill.

"All of us had two names," Mom had said. " I was never called Nelle. I was always Nelle Marshall."

The cousins all learned that family and kinship were not to be taken lightly. They have remained close to this day. After my mother graduated from high school, she enrolled in nursing school. It was during her nurse's training that she met my father, a young physician in training. Family was very important to her because her mother had died when she was 11 and her father lived several hundred miles away, so it was natural for mother to feel as if my father's parents were her own. Shortly after they were married, my parents went with my grandparents — PoPo and MoMo to me — on a fishing vacation to Leech Lake near Walker, Minnesota. It was my father's intent to introduce my mother to the wonders of a northern fishing experience.

They stayed in a resort where they were responsible for their own food and supplies. Mother was intrigued by the accents of the native guides, Jack and Dave, who doubled as house boy and iceman. She was wary of the Indian guides, but they all seemed friendly enough.

She loved the clear air with the scent of pine trees and was amazed that the clouds seemed so near. Everything was perfect until Dad informed her she would have to bait her own hook. She really could care less whether she had a minnow on her hook or not and finally enticed Jack to bait her hook when Dad wasn't looking. They had good luck trolling for walleyed pike over shallow reefs and had no trouble catching all they could eat.

One evening after dinner, my grandfather announced he had promised one of the Indian guides that he would stop down at the guide's tent and have a beer with them. My father was tired and he decided to hit the hay, so my grandfather took a pint of Old Crow and ambled out the door.

The next morning my father awakened early, and mother and my grandmother were fixing breakfast. PoPo was snoring loudly as he slept in his clothes on the cot in the front room. When he smelled the coffee, he got up and said, "Those Indians play a mean game of poker. I never saw so many wild cards."

He checked his pockets and had money in every pocket. He counted up and had $42. "Not bad," he mumbled and then checked his billfold. Instead of the three crisp $50 bills he had brought to pay for his vacation, he had only a Canadian $10 bill.

"They picked me clean," he groaned. His night at the Leech Lake Poker Club cost nearly $100.

Mother enjoyed visiting with Jack and hearing about his family and learning about their trials through the rugged winters. On their last day at the resort, Mother invited Jack and his family for a shore supper and Dad cooked steaks on the charcoal grill. It was apparent that beef was not a staple in their diet as they all cleaned their plates eagerly. Meeting new people from a different culture had been a thrill for Mother, a thrill she was to pass on to her own children.

Dad had hunted, fished and played golf with my grandfather all his life. They had been more than father and son, they had been best buddies. Their interests were the same. Dad did not want to get very far away from familiar territory, so after his internship and residency, he set up his practice in Ottawa, just 30 miles away from his hometown of Paola, Kansas. At every opportunity my parents made the trip to spend the weekend with PoPo and MoMo. Dad felt that the only way a person could really relax was to commune with nature, preferably with a fishing pole or shotgun in hand.

A creek that teemed with bullhead catfish and bullfrogs was across the road from the crude oil pump station my grandfather managed. Most weekends were spent bank fishing with cane poles with corks, worms or chicken liver as bait during the daylight hours.

I was born two years after my father began his practice. He wanted me to have his name, but he knew having two Bob Golliers in the family would be confusing. Mother was dead set against calling me "Junior." The cocker spaniel was named Junior, and I was given a Roman numeral II on my birth certificate and was nicknamed Bud so as to have my own identity.

One Saturday evening, my father, PoPo and Uncle Woody set limb lines and trot lines. Fried chicken was the Saturday night fare and then a poker game ensued while waiting to run the lines and re-bait the hooks at midnight. I remember thinking they would never stop playing poker. MoMo always had me sit next to her and she would show me a card and ask me to tell her what it was as she was unsure of her vision. "Whisper to MoMo, honey. Don't let the others hear you."

After running the lines, the fish would be cleaned and put on ice. The fishing party would then grab about four hours of sleep before running the lines Sunday morning. More bank fishing was in order, and then back to the boats to take the lines out.

MoMo really enjoyed the fishing, but her eyesight was a problem due to cataracts. PoPo thought he solved that when he discovered a cork in a bait shop that emitted a short whistle when a fish pulled on the line. He bought two for MoMo and tied them to her lines and off they went. My father was fishing down the bank a few yards from them and noted that MoMo kept setting the hook and pulling her line in without anything on it. As she threw her line back in the water with disgust, Dad noted the smile on PoPo's face as he puckered his lips and the short whistle escaped once again.

"You've got another one, Mommy," PoPo said. As she yanked on the pole, he said, "Oh, too late!"

Weekend fishing expeditions to visit PoPo and MoMo are among my earliest memories. I remember the poker games, the good food and the good time everyone seemed to be having. I could hardly wait until I was big enough to run the lines with the men.

Finally, when I was five years old, Mother gave her permission. I was really excited as I stepped into the small rowboat on a very dark night. PoPo sat in the front with a bright flashlight to search the bank for bullfrogs while my father rowed from limb line to limb line. I was sitting in the back trying to stay out of the way.

I could hear the rustle and splashing of a fish pulling on a limb line down the creek. We were not going to get skunked. I wondered how many fish we would catch. I prayed I would see a bullfrog. As a quick answer, Dad spotted a frog and PoPo held the light in his eyes and the frog seemed paralyzed as Dad rowed the boat to the bank. Suddenly, PoPo lunged at the frog and into the gunny sack he went.

Most of the hooks were bare, but we finally had some luck on our return to the dock on the far shore. We had three bullheads and then we lifted the trot line, which had been tied between two stumps. PoPo grabbed it and lifted it. Something was wildly pulling the line down about halfway across the creek. "The live perch is better bait than the chicken livers," PoPo said as we made our way along the trot line. We got to the fish, PoPo lifted him in — a plump three-pound bullhead. "That'll make pretty good eating."

PoPo re-baited each hook and we were ready to go back to the house. As we were nearing the dock, PoPo spotted a large bullfrog under a bush. Dad thought he could grab the frog if I could hold the light right in his eyes. The frog did not blink, but suddenly the whole world went topsy-turvy as both Dad and PoPo tried to grab the frog at the same time. We were all thrown out as the boat capsized. The only thing I remember is sitting on a muddy bank, shivering, while Dad and PoPo were trying to turn the boat back over. I had gone to the bottom of the creek, assuming the jelly fish float, remembering the instructions of my swimming teacher. When my father and PoPo stood up in the four feet of water, I was nowhere to be seen.

They both groped for me and finally PoPo grabbed my jacket and up I came, a baptized fisherman on my maiden voyage. I remember vividly the trip home that night. We left abruptly with hardly a good-bye to my grandparents, aunt or uncle. I was wrapped in a blanket between my father and mother, and I can remember a harsh tone of voice I had never heard from my mother.

"Bob Gollier, you've just got to be more careful!"

"Yes, dear."

The fishing weekends continued, but I was never very far from my bright orange life preserver.

FOUR

THE RULES were simple: You treated everyone in the family with respect. You did the best you could, whether in work or in play, and you never made the same mistake twice. The rewards were simple: Satisfaction in a job well done. Deviation from the accepted standards resulted in swift and uncomplicated discipline. My brother, Fred, was two years younger, and Janie was two years behind him. We all knew where Dad and Mom kept the yardstick and what it could be used for. A major error in judgment resulted in a trip to the bedroom to reason with Dad, yardstick in hand. There was no confusion, everything was understood. There was no need to do a lot of talking. On occasion, behavior modification was accomplished by constructive criticism.

One rainy day, Fred and I were building a tent with a sheet and two chairs in the living room, and suddenly I turned on Fred and belted him in the mouth and yelled, "Son-of-a-ditch!!" Mother came running and yelled, "Bud Gollier, where did you learn language like that?"

"From Dad," I said innocently. "When his gun jammed while shooting at a rabbit in a ditch the other day!" (In retrospect, I realize I may have misunderstood him.)

"You go right to the bathroom and wash your mouth out with soap!"

Then one day, Fred came bouncing in the back door and noticed the once-a-week housekeeper, LuBell, scrubbing the floor. Mother was appalled when she heard Fred say, "LuBell, what does 'fuck' mean?"

LuBell's chin dropped and she struggled to find words. Then she chuckled and said, "Fred, where did you ever hear a word like that?"

Fred said, "I saw it on the sidewalk, and it said 'Kilroy was here.'" Fred was off to the bathroom this time.

By the time I was four, Mother was ready to expand my social horizons. She was eager for me to meet new friends. A family she had met at church had a boy my age. His name was Larry Forsythe. His family lived about four blocks away, directly on the other side of the Ottawa University Campus, which was directly across the street.

Mother gave me directions one day, and I took off across the campus with Junior, our cocker spaniel, and the neighbor's cocker close behind. I knocked at the door at the appointed time. Larry's mother opened the door. Mother had schooled me in proper etiquette.

"Mrs. Forsythe, I'm Bud Gollier. I'd like to introduce you to Junior Gollier and Rags Lamb." Larry's mother was honored to be introduced like a queen to my companions.

Larry and I hit it off well and became fast friends. In preschool, we teamed for the first time. We patterned our partnership after the comic book characters, Henry the Chicken Hawk and Ollie Owl. Larry was shrewd enough to motivate me to carry out his devilish schemes, so he was designated Ollie Owl, since Ollie, adorned with a mortar board, was the brains behind the comic book escapades.

Larry's or Ollie's pranks were usually directed to teasing girls, almost always with the help of toads, bugs or snakes. I balked at handling the snakes with a shrug and a terse, "It was your idea." We sent screaming girls to the teacher numerous times and were quickly confronted with the command, "Bud and Larry, you march straight home this minute!! I'll be calling your mothers!!" We were not easily discouraged and would spend the rest of the day plotting a new adventure. We planned to enlist a lieutenant, Bill Hysom, in one escapade. Our plan was to let Bill on our team as a full partner. He would share in the fun and get all the blame.

Bill lived a half block from me. Larry walked across the university campus, and we walked to preschool together. Bill's house was on the way, and he would meet us at the corner. Three is naturally an uncomfortable number in any endeavor. Three people can never agree on anything. Bill had the deck stacked against him at all times.

Larry and I were not thrilled to see Bill always waiting

for us at the corner. He quickly fell into step with us, so we quickened the pace or slowed it, whichever would serve to remind him he was the interloper.

It was an early spring day when we set our trap. Bill was waiting on the corner as we crossed the street. "Hi," Bill said.

"Hi, Bill."

"Hi, Bill."

After a few steps, Larry pulled the box of earthworms out of his sack. "Bill, you keep these for us. We've got one for every girl in school."

"What are you gonna do with them?" Bill said.

"We're going to take turns putting them down the backs of their necks," I said.

"Not me!"

"What are you afraid of?" I quickly asked.

"Afraid your mommy will find out?" Larry said with a sneer.

"No, I'm not afraid of anything."

"We thought you'd want to be in our club. You keep the worms and we'll take turns," I said.

"What do I do?"

"We'll wait until after the story," Larry began. "Then we take our naps on our rugs. You are right next to Beverly Hobbs. You take one of the worms and quickly drop it down the back of her neck."

Bill looked at the box. The worms were wiggling around on top of the moss. They were big and firm, almost four inches long. I had picked them out of Dad's supply of night crawlers he kept in the old refrigerator in the garage. I had chosen the biggest and liveliest ones. I was proud of my selection. Bill's eyes were bright with anticipation.

"What do I do next?"

"Hand Larry the box," I said. "He's right next to Nancy Scott."

"Bud gets the box from me. His assignment is the Stevens twins."

"Both of them?" Bill asked in a voice filled with excitement.

"Bud thinks he can handle it," Larry calmly said.

"What will the teacher do?"

"You just pretend you're taking a nap. She'll never find the box."

The class began each day by reciting the alphabet, then we took turns going to the bathroom.

"Now, children, gather around for the story," Mrs. Bundy said. "We have another story about Dick and Jane."

"Oh, no, not Dick and Jane again," I thought. "They are a couple of real drags. They never have any fun. No bugs, no frogs, snakes or worms. Their days are full of nothing."

I wasn't really listening as Mrs. Bundy began the story. I was looking at Bill. He kept looking in the sack. I was afraid he would give us away. He couldn't sit still.

"Bill, do you have to go the bathroom?" Mrs. Bundy asked.

"No, ma'am."

"Then sit still."

"Bud, are you listening? Lie down on your rug. It's nap time." I lay down with my hand propping my head up so I could watch Bill. I closed my eyes so the teacher would think I was napping, then opened them just enough so I could see Bill and Beverly.

After five minutes, Bill made his move. He reached into the sack and pulled out one of the giant night crawlers. He got up on his knees and leaned over. Beverly was lying on her left side, her back to Bill. Bill reached over and then he sat down and looked at Larry and then at me. He was puzzled. I sat up. Bill pointed to Beverly's hair. It was shoulder length and hung past her collar. Bill looked at me. I shrugged. He looked back at Beverly, put the worm on her shoulder and lay back down with his eyes closed.

He quickly sat up, remembering he was supposed to hand Larry the box of worms. He looked over at Larry, but Larry had gone to the bathroom. He looked over at me as I was getting up to go to the bathroom. A look of awareness crossed his face. He looked quickly at Beverly; he had to get that worm back, but it was too late. Beverly rolled forward and the worm dropped down to her cheek. She screamed. Mrs. Bundy was at her side immediately. Beverly was in tears. Mrs. Bundy saw the worm on the rug.

"Oh, Beverly, it's all right. It's just an earthworm. Where are Larry and Bud? That's strange, they're not here. Bill, what do you have in that sack?"

She looked in Bill's sack as he started stuttering. "N-not m-meee. It wasn't my idea. B-Bud and Larry."

"Now Bill, don't go blaming them. They're in the bathroom. I'm going to call your mother."

"But-but-but-but ..."

"No buts!!"

Beverly ran to the bathroom and met Larry and me as we dried the tears of laughter out of our eyes.

"I know." She walked quickly past us.

Bill was talking excitedly to the teacher when we came back.

"What's wrong, Mrs. Bundy?" Larry asked innocently.

"You know very well what's wrong, Larry. Bill told me the whole story. I've called your mothers. They are waiting for you. School isn't over for another 15 minutes, but you two march straight home!"

We crossed the street. When we got to the corner, I looked at Larry.

"Don't you think we should wait for Billy Boy?"

"Yeah, I guess so. He was a real stool pigeon!"

We waited on the corner with our hands in our pockets. Bill crossed the street tentatively. He was on his toes with a slight crouch, prepared to break into a run at the slightest hint of trouble. When Bill got to us, he said apologetically, "I had to tell her the truth."

Larry and I looked at each other and broke out laughing. Bill looked relieved.

Larry looked at Bill and said, "Let's go. You did just fine." We put our arms around him and headed home.

We lived in a two-story brick home of Georgian architecture with a red tile roof. Ottawa University provided us with a playground big enough to play a near regulation game of "rough and tackle" football, which we preferred to play in grade school rather than the sissy game of touch football. When we chose up sides, the coin flip for first choice would determine the winner.

The first choice was always Ervin Lee Michel. Whoever got Ervin Lee won because he was a fearless tackler. Several ball carriers were known to simply stop in their tracks and throw the ball in the air when Ervin Lee lowered his head. We all learned the hard way. "I'll try anything once," I had said to Buzz Kelsey when he tried to call a play with me running around Ervin Lee's end.

The goal lines were the large elm tree at Eleventh and Cedar streets and the sixth elm down Cedar Street. The boundaries were the row of elm trees and the sidewalk to the girls' dormitory. The playground was also large enough to re-enact Picket's Charge at the Battle of Gettysburg, during the time Woolworth's 5&10 Cent Store was promoting Civil War memorabilia with uniform replicas.

Nights on our childhood playground were limited to rousing games of "Kick-the-Can." Occasionally we disturbed a couple of college lovers lying out on a blanket to observe the Milky Way or the North Star, or so I thought. This was before space was cluttered with various satellites, which have since become a more common excuse for students with amorous ideas. Our playground gave way to Dutch elm disease and progress as the university expanded and built a new girls' dormitory and a chapel.

Three blocks down Eleventh Street was the edge of town, and Rock Creek provided an opportunity to hike and explore. Small sunfish could be caught, but fishing Rock Creek was of no interest to Fred and me since we could go to PoPo's anytime to fish or walk the banks of Wea Creek in hopes of catching a glimpse of old "Double Hump," a bullfrog that lived just above the riffles. We would dream of catching him someday, but we were always more relieved than disappointed when we found him not to be in his usual haunts.

Rock Creek was always handy when it was time to collect leaves, insects or rocks for Scouts or a school project.

Childhood in Kansas helps one learn to be creative with leisure time. My childhood was spent during the pre-television era when reading, board games and tents manufactured in the living room were standard responses to Mother's comment that it was too wet to play outdoors. These simple tents were a setting for some adventure such as a conflict between pioneers and Indians. We would often relive the settling of the West, or the tents would be an imaginary bunker for a squadron of U.S. Marines as they defended Pork Chop Hill from the hordes of Chinese communists.

Although violent, these childhood dramas somehow seem innocent when compared to Dungeons and Dragons and other more modern fantasies inspired by computer games. Our fervor for the pioneer adventures was fueled by Mother's revelation that we were descendants of Daniel Boone, admittedly a very loose connection when reviewed with wisdom imparted by maturity and objectivity.

Fred had a passion for toads, and many of his playtime hours were spent in the basement window well of one of our neighbors where he kept every toad he could find. At one time, he had as many as 15 toads of all sizes and shapes in his collection. Fred was proud of his toad friends and even gathered them all in a barrel to show at the grade school carnival one year with a sign on the barrel — "Fred Gollier's Toads, a penny a peek."

One day when Fred was visiting his friends in the window well, our neighbor, a retired geologist, was in his basement and saw Fred. He opened the window and said, "Freddy, get out of there, that's where I keep my toads!"

Startled, Fred shot back, "Excuse me, sir, but they're my toads."

My little sister, Janie, was the belle of the ball from her birth and was a typical girl. She had a way of winning the hearts of all except her older brothers, whom she referred to reluctantly as "Boy" from the time she uttered her first word. By the time she was old enough to recognize we were, in fact, two different people with separate names, she was also old enough to tell she had gotten our goats. So, we remained "Boy" until our early teenage years; then she hardly spoke to us at all.

She had won our hearts, since we suffered with her when she battled her way back from polio at age nine. Her left leg was affected by polio, and she endured painful physical therapy exercises without complaints. The exercises helped build her muscles up. She was able to walk without her brace by the time she was in junior high. She worked hard at swimming lessons at the city park pool and earned the Red Cross junior lifesaving badge.

As a junior in high school, she became a cheerleader and was a leader in her class. She was thrilled when she was honored by her teachers and selected to go to Sunflower Girls' State. Mom and Dad were so proud when they took her to Lawrence for the week.

However, joy turned to tears when her call came that she could not stay because she had had polio. Fred went with Mom to pick her up; Janie was devastated! After all her hard work and pain, they were going to treat her like a leper. She was a cheerleader, a lifesaver, but she couldn't be a Girls Stater! Fred could not suppress his anger. As they walked out the door, he looked at the sponsor and said, "I suppose you voted against F.D.R."

Mother had come from a hotbed of New Deal Democrats, but she had turned tail after the Korean War and the specter of socialism during the Roosevelt and Truman years. Her main attraction to Roosevelt was his determination to overcome his disability.

"The time was right for him and the country. He saved the country after the depression," Mom had said.

The sixth member of the family was the cocker spaniel. He was epitome of man's best friend. Mother talked to him just like she talked to the rest of us.

"Time to eat, Junior."

"Don't do that, Junior!"

Junior lost an eye to infection as a puppy, and Mother was worried about him running into traffic. She called Uncle Marshall and Aunt Mary Pile, who had a farm near Marshall, Missouri, and they agreed to take Junior. Mother felt she had lost a child. After a week, the phone rang. "He's on the bus to come back to Kansas," Aunt Mary said. "He's chased all the cats to the barn and the hens won't lay. We can't keep him any longer."

Junior had free run of the neighborhood in the days before the leash law. Some days he would roam a little far and

Mother would get a call since her name and phone number were on his collar. "The cab will be there in a few minutes," she would say. In those days, Mother didn't have a car. "I would just call the cab and they would go get him for a quarter."

Junior repaid her loyalty when Fred crawled out into the street one day when he was a toddler. Mother thought he was on the front porch, and she was shocked to look out the front window and see Junior tugging at Fred's diaper in the middle of the street.

Mother was innovative for emergency babysitting help when she had an errand to run. It was down to the corner bus stop and a trip around town. It took 30 minutes and only cost a nickel per child. We were told not to get off the bus at our corner unless Mother was waiting for us. Mr. Burgoon, the bus driver, did not seem to mind. Mother always greeted him with a cheerful, "I hope they weren't any trouble." He never seemed surprised when we handed him an envelope at Christmas time.

I remember as a 13-year-old the annual Junior Chamber of Commerce Easter Egg Hunt at Forest Park. A few of the eggs had the name of a downtown merchant taped to them and could be exchanged for a prize if found. I lined up with the rest of children and took off at the sound of a whistle. I found six eggs, but none were endowed with the magic labels. Disappointed, I walked through town. As I walked past Robe's Hardware, Norman Murdock, a classmate, came out grinning.

"Hey, Bud, look at this neat pocket knife!" He showed me his fancy new Boy Scout knife, complete with a can opener, bottle opener, screwdriver and nail file. Then he said, "They didn't take my label. Do you want it?"

The temptation was too much. I took it off his egg and put it on one of mine. We decided it would be too much of a coincidence if the egg was the same color. Besides, his egg was smashed pretty badly. I walked into the store and handed Mr. Robe the egg.

"That's strange," he said. "They told me that they would only put out three eggs for me and this is the fourth I've received. Let me make a call."

He went into the office and I began to sweat. After what seemed like an hour, Mr. Robe came back. "There must have been a mistake. Here's your knife."

I walked to the door, turned around and called to him. "Mr. Robe, I took the label from the last kid who came in here. I'm sorry, here's your knife back."

"Young man, I want you to have this knife for being honest."

That evening I told my father about it, expecting him to congratulate me for being so honest. His only comment was a terse, "That's real poor." He couldn't have made a bigger impression with his yardstick. I had let him down.

I tried my hand at merchandising early. I had surprising success selling tickets to penny suppers at the grade school and chances on white elephant gifts at the Cub Scout booth at the carnival. Mother was my best customer, and she would buy my tickets for relatives and some of the neighbors. The near neighbors always seemed eager to buy from me.

When I traveled out of my territory, my product didn't do so well. I finally decided to move into seeds and magazines. The same people would seem interested at first and I placed a few orders, but it seemed like a lot of work. When the seeds didn't grow and the magazines didn't arrive, I knew it was a lot of work.

Since sales didn't seem to be my bag, I moved onto magic tricks. I sent for a catalogue from a magician's wholesale house in Royal Oak, Michigan, and received the promised free trick. It involved a reappearing coin that was dropped into a funnel that had a piece of glass at the bottom to keep the coin from passing through.

The trick was to make it appear as if the coin had passed through the funnel and to palm a second coin as the first was dropped through. And then presto, the coin reappears in the funnel as the great magician shows the audience the first coin that he dropped through the funnel and found in his hand.

I performed that trick at a Girl Scout meeting when one of their members was putting on a magic show. As I dropped the coin in the funnel, my hand hit the bottom of the funnel and the piece of glass and coin rolled to the floor. The room was filled with snickers and giggles as I sheepishly slipped the coin I had palmed into my pocket. That did it for my career as a slight-of-hand master in vaudeville.

Still in search of a profession, I went to the ads and it jumped out at me — taxidermy!! I eagerly filled out the coupon for a free instruction book as I enrolled in the Northwestern School of Taxidermy. I never heard from them. Perhaps they were discouraged by the age on my application form. I was smart at 11 and big for my age.

It looked as if I was going to have to stay in school. I just couldn't seem to get a job. Why couldn't I be as successful as Buzz Kelsey or Larry Prager? They were making a mint selling fireworks. Of course, they lived on Main Street and they had the idea first. They were in the "big time" and I was still door-to-door trying to sell garden seeds and zinnias. Buzz is now a successful attorney; Larry has been with Western Electric for more than 30 years. They have done well after their early successes.

I always enjoyed athletics. A basketball goal on the driveway provided many escapes into the fantasy life of big-time athletics during my early teens. I played many championship games on that driveway. Sometimes I imagined I was Bob Cousey, Bob Pettit or Oscar Robertson, but usually I was a Kansas Jayhawk. Jerry Waugh and Clyde Lovellette were the Kansas basketball stars of the late 1940s and early 1950s, and I followed them closely. I patterned my hook shot after Clyde, the center on the K.U. national championship team of 1952. I was thrilled when they went on to win the Olympic gold medal. Although I had never seen Clyde in person, I had read all accounts of the Jayhawk's success in the newspaper and had not missed one game on the radio. I felt I could visualize Clyde's hook shot in minute detail.

One day Fred and I were shooting baskets after school and having a rousing game of one-on-one. I suddenly looked up the driveway at a car that had just pulled in. The driver got out first and I recognized Art Jensen, a Kansas highway patrolman and a good friend of my father's. The passenger door opened, and the biggest man I ever saw got out, and as he stood, I thought he would never stop extending himself. They walked down to the basket, and I tossed the big man the ball and said timidly, "Mr. Lovellette, would you like to shoot a basket on our goal?"

"Sure," Clyde replied, and he softly ripped the cords with a gentle hook shot. I was the only one who knew he had made that same shot thousands of times on that same goal in a miniature body.

Art suddenly spoke up, "Boys, we've got to go. I just brought Clyde down to speak at the Rotary Club, and he is supposed to be at the meeting in five minutes. I promised your father we'd stop by for a few minutes."

Fred and I were stunned and speechless as Clyde bid us farewell with the advice, "You should get a jump rope and practice jumping rope every minute you can. That will help your reflexes, quickness and jumping ability." Then he and Art walked up the driveway to Art's car. It was a magic moment in the lives of two young boys.

There were obstacles in my march to fulfill the dreams that had been inspired on that backyard goal. One of the obstacles was my ninth grade coach. During a game with Emporia, a rival to the southwest, we were struggling and losing by a wide margin. I wasn't playing well. The coach was frustrated with the team's lack of success.

During the fourth quarter a loose ball was bounding toward the sidelines. I went after it and as it bounced toward the sideline, I grabbed it, turned and threw it back onto the court. I thought I had made a great save, but was chagrined to see an Emporia player scoop up the bounding ball and take it the length of the court for a lay-up. I stumbled and my fall had been cushioned by one of my teammates on the bench. I stood up after regaining my balance and was face to face with my coach. He looked at me sternly and said, "Gollier, you're as worthless as tits on a bull!"

As I walked home that night, all I could think about was the coach's comment, and I made a resolution to show him that he was wrong about me. I worked harder than ever on my shooting skills and took Clyde's advice and devised an area in the basement where I could jump rope. I got permission from Orlis Cox, the physical education teacher, to be excused from study hall so I could go to the track and run a couple of miles every day. Mr. Cox told me I had to learn to push myself. He talked of the difficulties in running a race: "A race is like life. There are times you must push yourself through the hard times. The quarter mile is one of the hardest races to run. At the far turn conditioning will pay off. It's like you hit a wall. You have to learn to run through the wall."

Mr. Cox had been in Ottawa forever. He had coached and taught physical education to the youth of Ottawa since 1923. He taught us to respect our bodies, follow the rules and to have high expectations in our physical endeavors. He continually asked us to run faster, jump higher and work harder. He taught us that laziness would beget laziness. His achievement tests in physical education were consistent with his philosophy. He graded on effort and improvement rather than on ability. Orlis coached football, basketball and track and coached several state champions.

In 1933, Orlis and his wife drove his state champion 880-yard relay team to Chicago to compete in the National Interscholastic Track and Field Meet, the last year for this championship. The Ottawa team was second in the preliminary heat, beaten by a Cleveland high school team with Jesse Owens running anchor.

The Ottawa team was anchored by Jack Richardson, who held the school record in the 100-yard dash. Clarence Heckroot, who had just won the 220-yard dash at the Kansas state meet, ran third.

Before the finals, Orlis met with his team at breakfast. "Boys, we're going to make a change. Clarence is a front runner, Jack will run third and should get us in the lead. I don't think Jesse can catch Clarence."

Just as Orlis had hoped, Jack had a three-stride lead as he passed the baton to Clarence for the final 220 yards. Clarence fulfilled the expectations of his coach as he broke the tape ahead of Jesse.

Mr. Cox did not limit his leadership and sense of fair play to physical education classes. As first director of the Ottawa

Recreation Commission, he implemented a comprehensive recreation program for youth as well as adults and the elderly. He left nothing to chance and planned for his program to be available to all citizens, particularly the underprivileged and minorities.

In the early 1960s he proposed that blacks and Hispanics be admitted to the segregated municipal swimming pool. Anticipating a storm of protest, he called a town meeting at the City Hall. My good friend and neighbor, Tom Gleason, was city attorney and gave me the following report. The storm gathered as anticipated, and Orlis gently opened the meeting by reading his plan for opening the pool to everyone. He was an imposing sight.

The audience numbered nearly 30. The majority of the crowd were young and middle-aged adults. They seemed to fit a mold. They were whispering among themselves, and their body language indicated they were on a mission. They were animated and could not sit still. Finally, Mr. Cox ended his opening remarks. "Does anyone have any questions?" Three people stood at once. Orlis spoke again, "One at a time."

A well-tanned man with a crew-cut raised his hand. One could not mistake the words "Stonewall" tattooed below the Confederate flag on his left shoulder. "Mr. Cox, I think things have been pretty good at the pool. The colored won't use the pool. They don't even like to swim." There was a rustle in the crowd with several audible murmurs of approval. Orlis looked up. "Thank you. Anyone else?" As the man sat down, there was a smattering of applause.

A young man stood up, but he looked nervous so he sat down. He then got up quickly and said, "They've got rights like anyone else. They pay taxes, too." He sat down just as quickly and looked down, not eager to meet the gaze from the man with the tattoo. Another man raised his hand. He had a notebook in his hand. He was sitting in the group with the first speaker. "Mr. Cox, I had an entire speech written out. I'm going to spare everybody the time. My kids use that pool. Their friends all learned to swim there. I hope my grandkids will learn to swim there. It's a well-run operation, a clean place, but it's just barely making its expenses. If you open the pool up to the niggers, the white kids will stay away." He then sat down.

Orlis pushed his paper aside. "You spared me your speech, I'll spare you mine. You say the Negroes don't like to swim. You say the white children won't swim with them. I guess we'll find out because it's time. The white boys and girls will still swim if you'll let them."

The meeting was over. The crowd filed out quickly. The man with the tattoo and his friends were the last to leave. As they left, the man with the tattoo walked up to Orlis. "Mr. Cox, thanks for letting me have my say. I hope it works out. We won't get in the way." Orlis looked at him and spoke softly. "I know it, Stonewall. Your dad ran for me in Chicago in 1933. He was a fair man. We've all got to speak up and make our point, then we put it behind us and move on. Good night, Stonewall."

"Good night, Mr. Cox."

My hard work paid off during my sophomore season. I played on the junior varsity basketball team and enjoyed a competitive high school career. Our teams didn't win any championships, and there were no scholarships coming my way, but we did win more games than we lost and we had the thrill of beating the eventual league champions on their home court both my junior and senior years.

I remember the Atchison game best. We had been beaten badly in our season opener the night before. Our coach told us to slow the game down and play with determination and patience. We kept the game close, and with less than a minute to play we were one point behind. An Atchison player took a short jump shot and missed. I lunged for the rebound, and an Atchison player grabbed my arm. The whistle blew with 20 seconds left. One and one. The cotton grew in my mouth as the referee handed me the ball. I looked at the rim. The noise was deafening. The Atchison pep band was blaring their fight song. I saw the bass drummer through the glass backboard. He made a face at me. I looked back at the rim. The gym became silent. The ball left my fingertips, not exactly a swish, but the game was tied! The next free throw was more artistic, and we hung on to win. I would have liked to have seen my ninth-grade coach after that game!

After high school, I went to the University of Kansas and received permission from Coach Dick Harp to walk on and play on the freshman team. The freshman team coach was Jerry Waugh, one of the idols of my youth. That was when I met the final obstacle in the pursuit of my dreams — limited ability.

After that year, I had the satisfaction of knowing I had gone as far as I could go in my basketball endeavors. Talent would take me no further. But that is what life is all about.

I knew that hard work and effort would be rewarded. The early years on the driveway had paid dividends. If one didn't push oneself to make the most of his ability, he would never know how far he could go.

FIVE

Autumn in the Midwest is a refreshing time. The stifling heat of August is replaced by cool, crisp mornings, and the leaves signal the end of their life cycle by turning a glorious array of colors. The greens are brighter as if they realize their days are numbered. The yellows, reds and oranges triumphantly announce the new season and seem to almost glow. The term "a breath of fresh air" must have had its origin on one of these mornings, when a sense of energy is imparted as Mother Nature warns us of a change in seasons. The weather changes also bring a sense of anticipation to fall activities. Football games and hunting season are on the horizon.

Quail hunting was another of my father's passions. He managed to hunt three days a week every hunting season. Fred and I were allowed to tag along and help carry the game at a very early age. Dad was very careful that we kept up with the hunters and never wandered ahead of or behind the guns. For Christmas at age 10, Dad gave me a single shot, 410-gauge shotgun, and I was allowed to carry it the next hunting season. However, I was not allowed to put a shell in the chamber until I was 12. We had done some clay pigeon shooting, and Dad had laboriously gone through gun safety with me. His philosophy was summarized in his frequently quoted rule:

"Never point your gun at anything you don't intend to shoot, never shoot anything you don't intend to kill, and never kill anything you don't intend to eat."

Good sportsmanship was the lesson to be learned along with safety. We enjoyed hunting with Dad's friends. Jim Frizzell came from St. Louis every hunting season. Merle Price and Art Jensen were local cronies who enjoyed pursuit of the wily Bob White quail.

None of Dad's friends loved the outdoors and hunting activity more than Cliff Haverty. Cliff was a fun-loving, ruddy-faced man whose curly hair had turned white. He owned a food market and did custom butchering. We would stop by the Zero Food Mart and pick Cliff up for the hunt. He would stick his head in the car and say, "Excuse me, I'll be right back." He would come back with two boxes of candy bars and gum, a box of apples and whatever else might be handy, like a carton of Coke.

He would say, "That ought to be enough, let's go get the dogs."

He kept the dogs that he and Dad shared in some sort of strange partnership. They had English pointers that numbered anywhere from one to seven over the years. All were capable, but a few were pretty rangy and were hard to control.

One day Cliff bragged to us about a new pup. "She has a heck of a nose, but tends to hunt a little wide." We let the dogs out, and Cliff's pride-and-joy took off over the hill — never to be seen again. Becky was one of our best pointers, but she had a tendency to be a little hard-mouthed and would occasionally eat a quail before finishing the retrieve, especially if the quail had been downed by my brother. Fred had been known to chase Becky a considerable distance before she turned and gulped the bird down just as he finally caught up with her. Quail was not Becky's only culinary passion. On one occasion, I caught Becky in a hen house and before I could get her out, four hens were lying on the floor of the hen house. Dad went to the farmer and paid for Becky's chickens, and we proceeded with the hunt. On another occasion, Becky bit off a little more than she could chew when she loped through a pigpen and killed a baby pig. By this time, Dad had seen enough.

"We have to fix that dog! I have a couple of ideas." One day Dad decided he would wrap a downed bird in barbed wire and have her retrieve it. Becky picked up the bird, looked at Dad with head slightly askew, spit the wire out and swallowed the quail.

"She's not so stupid!"

The next cure for Becky was a 50-foot length of rope tied to her collar to slow her down as she raced to the downed bird. It didn't slow her much, and Cliff finally said in his piercing voice, "I'll fix her!" As he quietly walked up to her, she was on point. He took the rope, tied it around his leg and said, "Bud, you go flush the bird, I've got the dog." A pair of quail exploded out of the fence row. I downed one and the other flew quietly away. I wondered why Cliff had not shot the bird, and I turned to find him flat on his back with Becky lunging and pulling his right leg with every leap.

"Untie me, Bud, this dog is incurable," shouted Cliff.

One day we were hunting with Hans Kuntze, an elderly farmer of Dutch-German extraction. He owned a section of land west of town. Hans, Cliff and Dad were walking up the road and Becky was hunting ahead of them. Suddenly a rooster jumped out of the ditch and set sail for the farmhouse about three feet off the ground. The rooster was making a lot of noise and was flying toward Dad and Hans. Becky turned her head and took out after the rooster. But the rooster had to go by Dad and Hans, and Becky was close behind traveling about 60 miles per hour. Dad was going to have none of that. He set his 280-pound frame directly in Becky's way. The collision was akin to the irresistible force meeting the immovable object. Becky went sprawling and Dad was flat on his back, and neither recovered very fast. The old German simply chuckled and looked at Dad and said, "Groundhog!" Later that day, Dad, Cliff and Hans were on one side of the thicket and I was on the other. As we walked on, the thicket widened and ran into a shallow ravine with a lot of dry leaves along the floor. I heard the quail running before I could see them. I then yelled at Dad, "About 40 of them on the ground between us!"

The quail ran on ahead and out into a meadow. Becky came in and we shot our limit with Becky making excellent points and Cliff, Dad and I shooting without a miss. Becky didn't even eat a quail. We went down to a stream and dressed out eight birds for our host. Dad said, "I was real proud of you, Bud. Hans couldn't believe you wouldn't shoot them on the ground. He said to me, 'You mean he sees them on the ground and won't shoot them?' I told him you wouldn't. I'm glad I was right."

Cliff gave me my first job. I worked at the Zero Food Mart the summer after the seventh grade. Dad assured me I was going to do something productive. Working for Cliff was more attractive than mowing yards. Cliff let me stock shelves, bag groceries and help in the meat market. It was my job to carry the waste to the back to be burned after butchering. Mother and Dad had a surprise birthday party for my 13th birthday. I bored all the guests by showing them my very first paycheck, which I had received that day — $14.27 for a week's work. I was really proud of that. My guests didn't seem impressed.

I grew up on the back roads of eastern Kansas. The search for the perfect spot to hunt or fish is endless. It will always be around the next turn, over the next hill or across the fence onto that farmer's land where permission is never granted. He didn't believe we were lost last year and he won't believe it this year either. Besides, Dad wouldn't hear of hunting without permission. To help the permission process, we always spent a day delivering packages of fruit cakes, candy and wine at Christmas time. Dad always knew exactly who was to get which package. There were to be no slip-ups!

When I started driving, the back roads were there to beckon me. We would begin the fall hunting season by sharpening our shooting eyes on the acrobatic turtle dove. Early mornings and late evening hours were the most productive. The doves flocked to feed and water at those times, and we would patiently wait for them to come winging in, always with the wind, and we never led them enough to hit them.

Since we knew so many likely hunting spots, Fred and I were always popular hunting companions. Larry Forsythe, my nursery school friend, had grown to be more than 6 feet, 5 five inches and was dubbed "The Big Turkey" by our basketball coach, speed not being one of his attributes. Turkey was always game for a hunt. When dove hunting, he always ended the hunt with a long face. One evening as we walked to the car, a single dove flew by us and landed on the corn stubble only 15 yards away.

"Take him, Turkey! Even you couldn't miss that one!"

Larry took aim with his grandfather's modified choke 12-gauge shotgun. Boom! The dust flew, and when it settled we heard the unmistakable beep, beep, beep of a turtle dove lifting in flight. The stunned dove flew erratically towards us, and Fred swung the barrel of his 410 at him, knocked him down and put him in his game pouch. Turkey just shook his head.

We were up before dawn when duck season opened. Going from pond to pond, we would sneak as quietly as we could to peek over the dam in hopes of catching a flock of ducks unaware. The best we could hope for was a long-distance shot and a prayer. Bruce and Bob Bundy were eager hunters. Bruce was Fred's age and Bob a year or two older than me. They were eager shooters, rather than hunters. When they walked through a section, nothing that moved escaped.

One crisp October morning, the sun was bright and the ducks and geese were moving in response to a frost moving into the Dakotas. It had rained several days before and the roads were all mud. We sneaked up on a pond, and a single mallard flushed out of the tall grass at the far end. Turkey raised his gun. Bob motioned him down.

"Turkey, he's 70 yards away." Boom!

The mallard splashed down like a Japanese kamikaze.

Bob looked at Turkey incredulously. "We've got to pattern that gun. I'm beginning to understand why you can't shoot doves."

We found a piece of paper and hung it on a fence. Turkey stood 20 yards away and took aim.

Boom!

The paper was gone.

"Turkey's got a cannon," Bob shrieked.

We then climbed into the car, a 1952 DeSoto sedan, and took off for the flats south of Homewood, 20 miles away. We were sliding from ditch to ditch, especially when the road ran out of gravel. A big flock of geese flew overhead. "They're looking for a place to land. Follow them!" Bob yelled.

"I'll try. They're tired of bucking the south breeze."

"Turn right at the next corner."

"I don't think the road goes through."

"Yes, it does. There's a low water bridge about a half mile down the road."

"It's awfully low. Probably be a quagmire with all the rain we've had this week."

The geese were getting lower and were just barely visible to the right. "Turn right!"

I did and went up a steep hill. I could feel the rear tires slip as we crawled up the hill. Hold her steady, I thought. Don't lose traction.

As I got to the top, my heart moved up into my neck. We were already heading down when Bob said, "Oh, my God, stop!"

"It's too late!"

The road was gone, the ditches were gone. There was water from fence post to fence post. With only the crown of the road intermittently showing to give us direction, I headed down. Keep the acceleration constant, keep your foot off the brake and keep the wheels straight! Not a sound from Fred, Turkey or the Bundys. A half-mile later we hit the low water bridge. The car didn't stall as we forded the stream. The road on the other side was graveled and we had good traction.

"That's the best piece of mud road driving I'll ever see," said Turkey.

We saw many flocks of ducks and geese that morning, but couldn't get close enough for any shooting.

We went home to eat. During dinner, the phone rang. I answered; it was Bob Bundy.

"Let's go out for a while this afternoon. You and I can sit in the car. We'll let Fred and Bruce run the ponds. If they see anything, they'll wave us on to help with the shooting."

"What if they don't wave to us and jump the ducks themselves?"

"We'll leave them."

"Sounds like it ought to work."

The day dragged on. No ducks. Fred and Bruce were losing their patience.

"Let's hit one more pond," Bob said. "The double pond at McCormacks. It's just a few miles."

We pulled in the gate and up along the fence. We were

just about to the crest of the hill when I saw them. Bob hit the brakes and ground the gears as he tried to jam the stick into reverse. I looked quickly back at the huge flock of Canadas, knowing they would be frantically beating their wings to get airborne, but they hadn't moved. It was as if they thought they were an exhibit at the zoo. We backed out to the road. Bob's cheeks pouched out like a prairie chicken starting to drum, then he giggled. Bruce was loading his gun. Bob took charge.

"Now, listen carefully! Bud and I will lead the way. We'll be in the middle. Fred, you're on the right, Bruce on the left. We'll crawl up to the base of the dam, and when we're all in position, I'll give the signal."

We all checked our guns and stepped out of the car. Bruce let his door shut. Bob gave him the look that the hangman gives the condemned men. The geese didn't fly.

We crossed the fence. I got stuck. Fred lifted the barb out of my jacket. Bob was already into his approach. He looked over his shoulder. We all quickly moved forward. Bruce started laughing, Bob started running. These geese didn't fly.

We were all moving fast. I watched Bob as he neared the base of the dam where we were to begin our assault. Bob was going to get the first shots. Fred realized it, too. We broke into a sprint.

Bob had two shots off and two geese down before I hit the top of the dam. I led a big honker as he left the water, his wing tips almost touching the water as I folded him up. Another shot and another goose fell. Then they were gone, circling above and honking to organize and continue their migration.

Fred and Bruce each had a kill, and we put the six geese in the trunk. There was no room for anything else.

We went back to town and showed our geese to our hunting friends. Turkey was in the bathtub. I routed him out with a story about the coyote we had killed. His expression of doubt indicated he knew me better than I thought.

"You really know how to rub it in," he said as he looked in the trunk.

Squirrel hunting was less enjoyable. I never got many

shots. You had to be quiet. We sat on a stump in a grove of trees for the longest time. Dad pointed to a tree and motioned me to walk around it. When I got to the other side, I could see him lift the rifle.

A sharp report and the squirrel came tumbling down. That was my role as a squirrel hunter — the noisemaker. It was impossible to walk quietly through the woods carpeted with dry leaves and brittle twigs.

Floating down the Marais des Cygnes River under the canopy of hardwood trees was a much easier way to hunt squirrel. Dad and I got into the rowboat with our .22's resting on our knees. The oars were in the oar locks, but the current would propel us at just the right speed. The wind was just a ripple through the trees. The smoke from Dad's Chesterfield was moving with us. I wished it would go away. Two squirrels were on the far bank as if they were playing tag. Up a hickory tree they went, one after the other.

They saw us and stopped. The boat moved on. Dad brought his rifle to his shoulder. Pow! Pow! A squirrel fell. The other squirrel crept around the tree trunk. I had him in sight, squeezed the trigger, but the safety was still on. I took the safety off. The squirrel was gone. I rowed over to the squirrel floating on the water. Dad put him in his jacket. We headed down the river. There was a noise in the trees ahead of us. A branch fell. I didn't see anything, but Dad did. He fired a quick shot. A gray squirrel fell to the water. Another squirrel in the jacket. Another Chesterfield!

SIX

MY INFATUATION with the far north was spawned in my youth on annual fishing vacations to the Lake of the Woods area in Ontario, Canada.

The summer vacations began when I was seven and our family would stay in a cabin on Lake of the Woods for two or three weeks. We journeyed north in the month of August every year until I went to college.

Jim and Charlotte Frizzell met us nearly every year. They were close friends of Mom and Dad and had been among their earliest friends in Ottawa. Their friendship had remained close after Jim and Charlotte had moved to St. Louis. They made their annual visit during quail season and always planned their summer vacations at the same time we scheduled ours at Mel's Canadian Camp.

Jim and Dad were like brothers. Their interests were exactly the same — fishing, hunting, cooking and eating. Jim preferred to fish with Charlotte and their daughter, Sally, and Dad always insisted his boat was filled with Golliers, but both boats fished the same water, and shore lunch was a group encounter.

One day Jim laid his rod down on the bow of the boat and began taking movies of our boat. As luck would have it, Mom picked up her movie camera and started shooting pictures of Jim as Jim turned and knocked his rod into the water where he could not recover it.

Several years later, while fishing the same reef, Dad hooked Jim's rod through one of the eyes and after pulling it in, he handed it to Jim, who was as usual only a few feet away.

Jim said, "You've got a fine touch, Buster."

Jim oiled his reel and fished the rest of the day with it.

Fishing provided most of the excitement, but we learned

one year Jim was not one to be dealt with lightly. Jim, Charlotte, Dad and Mom had gone to town for dinner one evening, and I decided I would demonstrate my newly acquired driving skills. I had passed my driving test a month before and had a restricted license. I offered to drive Fred, Janie and Sally to the Nestor Falls garbage dump to see the bears. We saw several black bears foraging around, and when we got back to camp, we met a different breed of bear. Jim was waiting for us and he was hot!

"You bit off a little more than you could chew, didn't you, 'Pretty Boy'?" Jim had called me "Pretty Boy" since I had been a toddler. I had never liked his nickname and I liked it less that night. I learned then that I was not old enough to make independent decisions.

The longing for the ultimate fishing experience had been bred indelibly into me. There was always the dream of a more desolate lake with fewer fisherman, perhaps unfished by man, and the promise of observing wild game in their native habitat, such as a moose in the lily pads, a deer swimming the lake or a bear in the blueberry patch. Our portage usually began at the Dog Paw Indian Reservation on the east end of Regina Bay on the Lake of the Woods. On our earliest trips, the portage was navigated by Dominic, the chief of the tribe. Dominic had a team of mules and he would back his trailer into the lake. Our guide would drive the boat onto the trailer, and Dominic would haul us over the portages, a one and one-half mile trek through the heart of the Indian village. Indian children were crawling on the trailer and riding along with us over the entire portage.

Over the years, Dominic's mules gave way to a tractor, and ultimately his business was taken over by one of his sons. The first lake on the other side of the portage was Dog Paw Lake, which was known primarily for its muskie. On every trip through Dog Paw Lake we would stop at Horse Shoe Reef and cast a few times to see whether we could raise a lunker muskie that inhabited the reef. We saw this muskie on a number of occasions, and it was a strange feeling to see him follow approximately 12 inches behind the lure and back off just as he was able to see the boat. There was a full six inches between his eyes, and my heart always raced when I saw that huge fish. I am uncertain as to whether I was hoping he would strike or hoping he would back off and leave me alone.

After Dog Paw Lake, we went through a narrows into Caviar Lake and then another tractor-trailer portage into Deer Lake, where we had fantastic walleye fishing. The four- to six-pound walleye caught in Deer Lake provided an unbelievable fishing experience, which is permanently etched into my mind. Cedar Tree Lake, a short portage off Caviar, was a haven for small-mouth bass. The bass fishing at Cedar Tree was discovered accidentally by Fred, who had been distracted after a slow morning of fishing at Cedar Tree one day, and caught two striped frogs during the lunch break. During the afternoon, he hooked one under the chin and brought in a small-mouth bass.

The next day we were back at Cedar Tree with a bucket full of frogs. We had no luck for a few minutes. I put on a Bass Master lure and threw it into a weed bed near shore. As I started to retrieve, I could see the water around the weed bed boil. I hooked a small-mouth bass and the fish — a four-pound beauty — suddenly leaped out of the water and assumed the pose that now graces the wall of my parent's family room. After we boated him, we caught fish, one after the other, until we ran out of frogs. By then we had enough fun and had kept only enough to eat, releasing the rest uninjured.

We were accompanied on our wilderness expeditions by our native guide of several years, Bill Brough, a former game warden who had a trap line in the winter and had enough stories to make even a fishless day exciting. Bill was a sturdy, good-humored man who was part-Indian and whose skin gave away the exposure to extreme weather. He had an unmistakable gleam in his eye, which betrayed the devil in him. You did not doze while trolling for walleye in Bill's boat as he would be tugging on your line in a manner that had been perfected to mimic the strike of a hungry fish.

At the end of each summer vacation, we would have a picnic with Bill's family. One year, near the end of our vacation, we had a very stormy day. Bill came to our cabin early for a cup of coffee. Dad had decided the lake was too rough to go out, but Bill insisted.

"I'll take Bud and Fred to an isolated bay where I have seen some lunkers through the ice while trapping in the winter."

That was all it took! Fred and I had our storm suits on in a flash and practically ran to the dock. As we started out of the protected bay onto the lake, which was topped with rolling whitecaps, I looked under the tarp in the bow of the boat. My heart leaped as I saw two high-powered rifles. Bill had always talked of having venison steaks for our picnic, and today would be the day. Many times he had promised to take us deer hunting. We went up the lake about five miles through the rain and wind. Bill knew the tricks of poaching, and I sensed this was not Bill's first out-of-season hunt. He had learned how to feed his wife and four children on meager wages.

Bill instructed us to be very quiet and follow him about 10 paces. He wisely decided that he would be the only one to carry a gun. Off we went through the tall spruce and birch trees along a well-worn game trail. Bill pointed out tracks, bear droppings and deer droppings and gave us a real lesson in tracking. We quietly trudged on. After about two hours, Fred and I lagged a bit farther than the prescribed 10 paces behind. Bill suddenly turned and his eyes were widened with a real terror! He ran frantically toward us and shouted at the top of his voice, "Bear! Bear!!" My memory is indistinct as to whether he violently shoved us down or jumped over us, but he was by us in a breath, and as I collected myself for the mad dash from sure death, I looked down the path and Bill had suddenly disappeared around a turn. As Fred and I rounded that turn, Bill was sitting on a log and laughing uncontrollably.

It started to rain and we went up a small hill. I could see a marshy bog through the trees, and Bill suddenly stopped. I heard a noise and Bill's gun went to his shoulder. There was a flash of color to our right and a crash as we had jumped two does out of a thicket and they bounded to the game trail to make their escape. One stopped suddenly and looked up the trail at us. I waited for the rifle's report, but none came. The deer trotted down the path, and Bill turned and said,

"Couldn't get a shot off." I knew better. He had known we were four miles from the boat, and lugging a deer that distance, with two young boys, was going to be quite a chore. Bill was not about to leave the meat to spoil, and he had decided that the risk was too great. I had no question that had Fred and I not been along, that deer would have been a goner.

There was always talk of fly-in fishing trips to remote lakes, and our family made a number of trips either via float planes or primitive portages where we went from portage to portage across in-between lakes on whatever boats we could find. Bill would always say he had checked with the natives and that boats would not be a problem, but they always were a problem. We usually had a choice of two leaky tubs, and it was a matter of the lesser of two evils. If there was a decent boat available, another party would arrive at the same time and claim it. My father was not very persuasive or argumentative and always let the others have their way; after all, he was on vacation. As I think back on it, I am surprised he never rattled about the lousy boats we always had on those trips. My father could not swim. We had some great fishing experiences on those remote lakes. In addition to Cedar Tree Lake for small-mouth bass and Deer Lake, there was Rowan Lake for walleye and High Wind for lake trout. It was always an adventure, and there were always dreams that the next cast was going to bring "Daddy Warbucks" out of the depths.

It was always exciting to see wild game in their native habitat. Moose, deer and bear were plentiful. There was always talk of Great Bear Lake and Great Slave Lake up on the Arctic Circle. That was my ultimate dream, just to get up there for one short week and have a chance to catch monster trout casting on the surface. The owner of the resort was Mel Carpenter, and he was planning to build a fishing camp at Great Bear Lake and was always talking about his fabulous fly-in fishing trips. When I was in college, I wrote him and asked for a summer job after his camp opened. To my surprise, but not to the surprise of my father, he wired back and agreed to hire me as a fishing guide. He knew I had had a good apprenticeship. It was much later I discovered Dad had laid the groundwork for me.

When Dad convinced Mel to hire me as a guide at his camp on Great Bear Lake, my dream was beginning to materialize. The summer before my first year of medical school, I traveled to Winnipeg in early June. I followed Mel's instruction as I crossed the border.

"Don't tell them where you will be working as I can't get you a work permit. Whatever you do, don't tell them you're an American."

The Canadian customs official looked very uncomfortable in his well-pressed navy blue uniform.

"Where are you going?"

"Fishing up north."

"Where are you from?"

"Ottawa."

"Oh, you're going home after the holiday?"

"Yes, sir."

"Very well. Have good fishing."

"Thank you, sir."

The southern boundary of the Northwest Territories is the 60th parallel at 60 degrees north latitude. Part of the spirit of the hardened native is manifested in the term "North of Sixty," the slogan of the Northwest Territories. "North of Sixty" is usually seen on souvenirs with the polar bear logo that has long represented the Northwest Territories. The phrase "North of Sixty" is used by those who understand the reality of the long, cold winters with nearly constant darkness. Inside the Arctic Circle, the sun does not rise above the horizon on December 21, while those in the capital city of Yellowknife enjoy five hours of daylight. The dawns and dusks are longer than one might think because the sun sets at such a low angle and the days are blessed with extreme day-long periods of twilight. Those from the south can only imagine the planes on skis, the tractor trains over the ice and the caribou hunts with snowmobiles driving the caribou into the Indians' guns. There is a sense of pride and accomplishment seen in the natives' weather-thickened, expressionless faces. They are fixed as if they would shatter if a smile accidentally crossed their faces.

I arrived in Winnipeg and made connections at the Airport Hotel. I was given a briefing by Bud Williams, the personnel manager, and was introduced to the other guides. There was an equal mix of young college students from Kenora, Ontario, and seasoned native guides from the Sioux Narrows area around Lake of the Woods. We had more than a few beers and got acquainted. I quickly became "Kansas" and learned everyone's nickname. There was Huck, Moe, Chico and two Killers — Killer I and Killer II, who were brothers from Kenora, Ontario.

The next morning we boarded the DC-3 for the flight to Great Bear Lake. We had a brief stop for fuel and supplies at Yellowknife before continuing on to Saw Mill Bay on the shore of Great Bear Lake, 200 miles farther north. At Saw Mill Bay, there was an old RCAF Dew Line sand airstrip that was 20 miles from the fishing camp. The sand airstrip was composed of soft sand and provided very exciting takeoffs and landings. As we neared Great Bear Lake, I was really excited. I kept my eyes on the horizon and asked myself the same question as a new body of water came into view: "Is that Great Bear?" When I saw it for the first time, the question did not need to be asked. Suddenly the plane banked slightly and turned to the left a few degrees. I was astounded to see my first view of Great Bear Lake, 200 miles of unbroken ice. I couldn't believe it! All the guides were hooting. "They sent us up a week early to be bloody ice breakers," came a shout from the back of the plane. As we descended on our approach to the Saw Mill Bay Airstrip, I would see the ice was beginning to break up into large flows and there were occasional patches of open water. What was in store for me? I could tell it was going to be an exciting summer!

As the DC-3 slowly ground to a halt on the soft sand airstrip, I wondered how it could ever obtain enough speed to get airborne again. The steward explained they always took off with a much lighter load and the runway was long enough, so there was no problem getting off the ground. We unloaded the baggage and supplies from the DC-3 onto the ground so it could be loaded into an amphibious aircraft, a large-bellied Grumman Goose. There was just enough open water in the bay behind camp for the Goose to land and take off as it could get airborne in a very short distance. We had an unusual problem with the first load to camp. The Goose got mired in the sand. The camp foreman excitedly yelled at us, "That plane's stuck. You guides go push it out!" Talk about a new experience!. All I could do was shut my eyes for protection from the blowing sand and grab a door or wing strut and rock the plane until it gradually began to inch forward. Soon the plane was off. The DC-3 got off quickly, and I had nothing to do but wait because the Goose was the only transportation available.

Usually most supplies and personnel were transported by boat, but the ice made that impossible. As we approached the camp, I was astounded by the beauty of the area. On the left was a large mountainous island marked by rocky outcroppings of the pre-Cambrian shield, composed of ancient igneous rocks. The rocky outcroppings were separated by strands of evergreens, birch and poplars that grew out of the muskeg in the moist hollows and thicker stands of spruce and evergreens that populated the lake edge. I could see the camp in the distance with the white cabins and bright red roofs sitting on a peninsula out into the narrows. There were large beautiful cliffs on each side of the inlet, and I saw the wreckage of a small plane strewn along the rocky face of the island. This served as a monument to the perils of the country.

"He was on skis last winter," the pilot, a David Niven lookalike, shouted at me. "He didn't have as much runway as he thought he had. There is no way to stop them. You can only turn or take off again."

The first week in camp was all work. I was a painter, carpenter and plumber all at once. The worst job was digging the septic tank in the permafrost, which had the consistency of clay and begins 10 inches below the muskeg, which covers the ground between exposed rock.

The camp foreman was a raw-boned giant of a man named Hi Loomis. Ironically, Hi had previously owned a camp on Caviar Lake and our family had stopped by for a cup of coffee years before when fishing with Bill Brough. Hi seemed to be everywhere and was always stopping by the bunkhouse to see whether any of us were shirking duty. Moe Turcott, a guiding veteran of many years, became our watchdog. As soon as Moe opened the door to the bunkhouse and entered, Moe would say, "Sky-Hi is looking for you. Here he comes."

Hi was friendly enough, but there was work to be done and he darn sure was going to get it done. He did not ask anyone to work harder than he worked, but he always had an idea if a guide thought he had a day off when his party took one of the side trips to the Arctic Ocean to see the Eskimo community at Coppermine or to fish for Arctic char at the Tree River. Arctic char are beautiful fish and make a mad spawning run into the rivers flowing from the south into the Arctic Ocean. When Bill Murphy caught the world record char in 1962 and brought it back to camp, everyone was clamoring to make that trip. The guides usually didn't get to go, and at first that was perceived as a perfect day off and an opportunity to catch up on needed rest. Hi found Moe in the bunkhouse one day when his party went to the Tree and had him clean latrines all day. That night Moe said, "If you put a bolt in his forehead, he would look just like Frankenstein!" We all laughed ourselves to sleep that night, all but Moe.

The first fishing party was scheduled in five days, but with the ice conditions, I didn't think they would be a very happy group. On the third day, I was standing on the point in front of the lodge admiring the beautiful scenery at 11 o'clock at night; the sun was still high in the northern sky. I listened to the sounds of the ice as it moved slowly through the narrows between our camp and Richardson Island. The ice floes were huge and the evening breeze off the ice made me wish for a down parka. It seemed the ice would be there all summer. One morning while walking to the dining hall for breakfast, I noticed the ice had totally disappeared during the night. The wind had blown the ice north, and there was nothing but open water surrounding the camp. The guides were all assigned boats, motors and shore lunch boxes, but no one said anything about fishing. I wondered where to fish and what methods to use. The guides were not going to be any help. They weren't going to share secrets; it was going to be a competitive summer. Everyone just smiled and acted smug. The bosses didn't have any information either.

They just gave all the guides a map and said there were lures for sale in the camp store. It was apparent I was going to have to learn the ropes on my own. The Canadians all wanted to see what this American could do.

The first two weeks were really slow. I was feeling my way around, and I am sure I did not inspire the confidence of my fishermen, as I was constantly referring to my map, changing trolling speeds and moving to a different depth of water. All the guides were new to Great Bear Lake, and the veterans resorted to a basic fishing principle by fishing the drop-offs. This was easy enough to do as the clear water provided distinct demarcation between the dark blue of deep water and the lighter blue-green of shallow water. My tactic was to vary the speed of the motor while trolling in a zig-zagging pattern along the drop-off with frequent casts into the shallow and occasionally a cast out to the deeper water. I felt I had the greatest opportunity to attract a feeding fish by varying the conditions of water I fished. My boat caught enough fish to keep it interesting, but one of the other guides always had a bigger day. Every day someone had a 30- or 40-pound lake trout and I was doing well to bring in a dozen fish a day. The guides were razzing me all the time.

"What's wrong, Kansas? Not as easy as you thought, is it?"

Moe was the most help as he taught me to make a delicious fish chowder that has since become a Christmas Eve ritual at our house. After two weeks, I felt I could do everything I needed, but I was still unable to have a really successful day fishing. Huck Hanton was the most relentless in giving me a hard time. He was a wiry veteran guide, nearly toothless and was determined to boat the biggest fish each week.

"That's how you get a big tip," Huck said. "Catching the shore-lunchers won't do you any good; it has to be a real trophy."

One evening Huck said, "Why don't you follow me tomorrow, Kansas?"

I was willing to try anything, so the next morning we left the dock together and started fishing on the same shore. Fishing the drop-off, I was 100 yards behind him. My party of two was from Montana and had done a lot of stream fishing. One of them was continually urging me to move closer to the bank. He was inspired by the inviting rocks and shallows.

"We're not fishing for rainbow trout," I told him.

"Get in a little closer," he insisted.

I could see Huck looking back at me and smiling. We caught only four trout all day and Huck caught about 40, including a 32-pounder. He was merciless that night.

"What were you after, Kansas, rock bass?"

Things slowly picked up as I gained more experience. My charges boated a number of 20-pounders and one weighed 27 pounds, but the real trophy still eluded me.

After meeting the plane returning from Tree River each day, I became aware of a longing within me, and the humor of it did not escape me. I had finally arrived at Great Bear Lake, the dream of my youth, and it was not enough. Boating 20 to 30 fish from 10 to 20 pounds each day would not end my search. The quest for the ultimate fishing experience is never satisfied. Now the Tree River was there to haunt me, the Tree River and White Eagle Falls.

Fishing for lake trout tended to be a bit tiring. For variety, we had the opportunity to fish for Arctic grayling, a beautiful sporty fish with a large dorsal fin that inhabited the shore line and the tributaries to the main lake. The spinning rods and fly rods offered a change in technique that most fisherman enjoyed, in addition to the change in scenery. Approximately 30 miles from camp, the Camsell River emptied into Great Bear Lake from the south. At the wide mouth of the river the current was slow, and as we traveled upstream and the river narrowed the current became swifter.

After several days of trout fishing, most people were ready for a change of pace and were ready to go to the Camsell for grayling fishing. Approximately 10 miles upriver there were rapids, and several of the guides found that by emptying their boats and having their guests walk along the path around the rapids they could get up enough speed to bounce over the rapids and then fish above the rapids and on up the Camsell River to the next rapids, which were even swifter. Several of the guides, including me, were apprehensive about shooting the rapids, and the anxiety was increased when Bob England capsized his boat trying to shoot the second rapids. Huck considered himself "King of the River," but even he couldn't make it up the second rapids.

"It's just too rough, too many rocks," he said. "I don't think anyone could make it." On my second trip to the Camsell, Huck was along with the party ahead of us. I watched him run at the rapids and bounce over the first wave, then slowly regain his momentum and plane up into the smooth water above. I unloaded my boat and started out into the lake to build up speed. As I hit the first wave, the bow of my boat veered to the left, and as I hit the water a huge spray filled my boat with water. With all that unexpected weight in my boat, I was unable to gain any momentum and simply settled into the rushing waters, neither gaining or losing ground. I attempted to reach my coffee can to bail the boat, but it was too far forward. I also tried to pull the plug to drain the boat, but because I did not have enough speed, the water would not drain. I put the plug back in rapidly and slowly eased off the throttle and with a prayer backed out of the rapids. Luckily I was able to turn the boat quickly and run down stream out of the rapids over the first big wave. I then pulled the plug and drained the water out of my boat. As I went over to the shore, Huck grinned at me and said, "Pull your boat over here, Kansas, I'll run it up for you."

"No one is going to run my boat up those rapids!"

I took another run at it and this time kept the bow heading upstream after bounding through the first wave, and I was able to gain momentum and pull up over the rapids. The grayling fishing was excellent in the second rapids as we fished it. I was impressed with the violent turbulence of the water and could understand why Huck had said no one could run a boat up those rapids.

My next party was from St. Louis. Bill Cady and Jay Henges expressed early in the week a desire to camp overnight and to do some grayling fishing in unfished waters. Bill got the map out and ran his finger up the Camsell River. His finger stopped suddenly at White Eagle Falls just above the second rapids.

"I would like to fish here."

"It's inaccessible. Two guides tried to shoot the rapids below it. One swamped and the other said it was too rough."

"Let's go up there and camp and have a look at it."

After fishing lake trout for several days, we packed a tent, camping supplies and took out for the Camsell River. The first rapids were no problem, and we enjoyed fishing below the second rapids. We walked along the path to a high point and looked at White Eagle Falls. It was an imposing sight! A half mile away, I could sense the power of the rapids below it as I realized that all the water coming down White Eagle Falls also had to go through those rapids as there was no other escape.

From this elevated spot, I had a good view of the rapids. The water was smooth at the top and then tumbled down into a narrowed turmoil of white water. Suddenly I noted a deep-blue ribbon of smooth water along the far bank. That meant deep water. I could see the secret was to bear left after entering the rough water and to avoid the turbulence caused by the rocks and the shallow water.

That night we camped below the second rapids, and after dinner we were sitting around the camp fire with the roar of the rushing water in the background.

"I don't know if I can make it," I said.

"I thought the motto of all Kansans was 'Ad Astra per Aspera,' to the stars through difficulty," teased Jay. "Well, I guess tomorrow we'll find out," was my weak reply.

The next morning I had a knot in my stomach as the boat gained speed making a loop in the water below the rapids. I said a brief prayer as I approached the rushing water. The first wave was a huge crest, but my momentum took me through and over it with little problem. I veered left and was suddenly swept even farther left than I had intended and was concerned about being washed on shore. Suddenly my boat began to gain momentum as I hit the smooth water. As I topped the crest of the rapids and could see White Eagle Falls right in front of me, I knew that meeting that challenge was going to make future obstacles easier to overcome in the rest of my life.

"Nothing to it, Kansas, mind over matter," said Jay with

a smile as I steadied the boat for him to climb in.

Our fishing was all we had dreamed. We caught an uncountable number of grayling in the swift waters of the bottom of the falls, and the fight in the fish was enhanced by the leverage they gained with the huge dorsal fin in the fast water. At that time the world record grayling was four and a half pounds. We didn't have a scale with us, but several of our fish measured as long as the world record fish. I had never had a more exciting experience and could hardly wait to get back to camp to tell the other guides that I had made it to White Eagle Falls.

As we arrived at camp the next evening, my enthusiasm was quickly dampened. Mel Carpenter met us at the dock and said that Hi Loomis and Huck Hanton had picked up a load of airplane gas at the uranium mine at Port Radium, 40 miles north — almost exactly on the Arctic Circle. They had been expected back the same evening, but were 36 hours overdue. The mine was closing down and they had a cache of airplane gas that Mel had bought at a bargain price. It was assumed that the rough water had swamped their boat with the heavy load. It did not seem like the proper time to share the excitement of my trip to White Eagle Falls. The mess hall in the dining room was totally quiet. Everyone knew that any of us could have been in that boat with Hi; it just happened that Huck had gone along because his party was up at Tree River that day.

I never prayed as hard as I prayed that night.

The next day we all fished the shore between camp and Port Radium. I was looking for a cushion, a sign of gas on the water or a waving hand from the shore.

Two days later, our prayers were answered. The Mounty Air and Sea Rescue Team had found Huck and Hi in their boat floating out in the middle of the lake out of gas. One of their gas tanks had been filled with fuel oil instead of mixed gas, and when they changed tanks their engines suddenly stopped. When they got out of the plane at the dock, amid all the cheers of the guides and guests, I gave thanks that my prayers had been answered. To be reminded of the fragility of human beings in such a beautiful setting put things in perspective for me. Never had I felt the presence of God so strongly. By the middle of August, fishing had slowed considerably, and one week fishing was so poor the guests had complained bitterly to Mel Carpenter. He called a guides' meeting and instructed us all to save every fish we caught.

"I promised each guest 75 pounds of fish fillets, and we don't have one fish box full yet. I want you to save every fish so we can fill those fish boxes. I know a lot of you like to just keep the bigger ones to fillet, but we are going to need everything we catch."

I tried every place I could think of to find the fish. I knew lake trout spawned in the fall, and I thought perhaps the fish would be back in the shallow bays and areas we had fished early in the spring. But nobody was having any luck.

With just two days to go in the week, things were getting pretty testy. We had had another slow day, and I was fishing with a man and his wife from Iowa. They were part of an insurance company party, and their entire party was pretty disappointed. At 4 p.m. I decided to try one last place before dinner. We were traveling across open water to the reef I had in mind when I saw the gulls. About 40 sea gulls were diving at the water a quarter of a mile from shore. It hit me all at once. The lake trout were driving the ciscoe, their primary food fish, to the surface and the gulls were after the ciscoe. We sped out there quickly. I told my guests, "Throw your spoons out there and let it sink to the bottom."

The next 45 minutes were among the busiest of my life! We caught fish nearly every cast, from 7 to 14 pounds each. I remembered Mel's order, and we kept all that we caught. I have no idea how many fish we had, but the boat was loaded when we finally quit in order to be back at the lodge at the appointed time of 6 o'clock. However, with the load it took us much longer than I thought to make the return trip.

Six o'clock was a strictly enforced time at camp, and if anyone was late, everyone would gather at the dock to determine whether a search party should be sent. We could see the crowd at the dock as we approached camp. As we pulled into the dock, Mel Carpenter smiled as he looked at the fish in our boat.

"Huck, you and the guides come down and look at the fish in Kansas' boat. This is the way a real guide does it!"

Huck looked at me with a genuine smile and said, "You finally got lucky, didn't you, Kansas?"

Huck's smile faded as Mel looked at him and said, "Mr. Hanton, you and the rest of the guides are going to clean Kansas' fish this evening."

Huck and I walked out of the fish house at 10 p.m. after four hours of filleting fish with only a 10-minute break for a quick sandwich. As it was late in the summer, we were beginning to see a few hours of real darkness. The sun had set in the north and the stars were starting to make their presence known in the twilight.

"Let's stop by the camp store, Kansas, I want to buy you an ale," said Huck.

"Sounds like a deal!"

Huck went in and ordered two bottles of O'Keefe's ale. We went out to the dock and sat down in Huck's boat.

"You've been better than I thought you'd be, Kansas. You pull your weight."

"It's been a good summer. We didn't make a lot of money, but hard work is its own reward."

Suddenly I became aware of the glow above us.

"Aurora borealis," I mumbled.

"What'd you say?"

"The northern lights. They are really vivid up here. Look at the greens and even some deep reds! The light seems to pulsate. Look at it move!"

"Haven't you ever seen them before?"

"Not this close. Huck, look carefully. You know the lodge faces true north, that means the northern lights are southeast of us."

We were both captivated by the flickering waves of color. It was as if someone was waving a brilliantly shaded transparent sheet. There was no wind, but the sense of the movement demanded our attention.

"Listen to the lights!" said Huck.

"Are you crazy?"

"Listen close, my grandmother would tell me. She grew

up on the Bathin Island in the Arctic. She once said, 'Huck, listen to the lights. They are like boys playing ball. They chase each other across the sky. The sound you hear is the joy of their play.' "

Then I heard it! It sounded like a deep hollow whistle or a hum. The sound came in waves ever so faintly, but with the same rhythm as the waves of light.

It was a beautiful display, almost a symphony. It was a fitting final celestial aria to my summer North of Sixty.

We finished our ale and headed to the bunkhouse.

"Thanks for the ale, Huck."

"Good night, Kansas. It's been nice knowin' ya!"

SEVEN

". . . I will prescribe regimen for the good of my patients according to my ability and my judgment and never do harm to anyone. . . If I keep this oath faithfully, may I enjoy my life and practice my art respected by all men and in all times, but if I swerve from it or violate it, may the reverse be my lot."
— Hippocratic Oath-

"ANYTHING WORTH DOING is worth doing well." That was my physician father's standard reply whenever Fred, Janie or I didn't quite measure up to his expectations in the classroom, on the athletic field or in any task we set out to accomplish. It was his philosophy and legacy and his patients got the message. They knew he cared, was always available and always had their best interest foremost in his mind.

Dad decided to be a doctor at the urging of his father. PoPo had worked hard to help his younger brother through medical school, and he encouraged Dad to follow the same path. He told Dad that if he studied hard to become a good doctor, perhaps he could find time to hunt, fish, play golf and enjoy the type of life he had provided him without the sacrifices they had to make. Dad worked hard at his studies at the University of Kansas, but it did not come easy for him the first semester. He was relieved when the Christmas break came and looked forward to hunting rabbits with my grandfather over the holiday. They had a nice visit the first night home. The next morning my grandfather rudely rolled Dad out of bed at 5 a.m. Dad could hear the horn honking in the driveway over the howl of the winter storm.

"Get dressed, Buster, that's the Pipeline truck!" I got your down slips from the University yesterday. You have a two-week job with the pipeline, and if you don't start studying, you can do that for the rest of your life."

My father never had another down slip.

I was determined to be a doctor like my father. When we were very young, he would awaken Fred and me to go on house calls in the country. We would doze off in the car while he was attending the patient or delivering a baby.

One night we were awakened by the slamming of a trunk. Tony Plaschka walked around from the back of the car with Dad.

"Thanks for coming out, Doc, Liz and I sure 'preciate it!"

"You're welcome, Tony. The penicillin should start to work in a few hours. I'll be back to check her tomorrow evening."

Dad drove the eight miles back to town quickly. The gravel made a deadening sound on the under-belly of the car. As we drove in the driveway, the headlights revealed the basketball goal and the white picket fence next to our garage. As we got out of the car, Dad said, "Either of you boys got a test tomorrow?"

"Uh, huh!"

"No, sir."

"How'd you like to learn how to skin a guinea?"

"All right!!"

"You bet!"

Suddenly I realized that Dad and Tony had put his payment in the trunk.

We were proud of Dad. He loved his work. He felt it was very satisfying, but he was terribly frustrated by tragedy. When a patient developed an incurable disease, it affected him for weeks. He had a very difficult time with his failures. He was frustrated when he could not alter the natural course of things. During the polio epidemic of the early 1950s he suffered with the families of every victim. His frustration hit a high point when Janie had a headache and fever. Dad did the spinal tap in her bedroom. The laboratory confirmed his fears — she had polio. She was an inspiration to others in her recovery. A slight limp was her only affliction, and she made people unaware of that by keeping them off guard by always asking about their problems and being interested in other matters. That response did not soften the blow to my father. When he had bad news to convey, it was written all over his face. My first personal confrontation with death occurred when I was 15. Our next door neighbors were just like family to us. Harold and Blanche Lamb — Uncle Harold and Aunt B to me (no blood relation) — had made us welcome when we first moved to their neighborhood. In early childhood, I could always sense when Aunt B was pulling cookies out of the oven, and she never seemed to be too surprised by my knock at her back door. "Why, Bud, what a pleasant surprise! Come in dear, I just happen to have some cookies." One evening I stopped to visit with Uncle Harold. I sat down at their dinner table. As he was finishing dessert, Aunt B happened to have another piece of pie.

"Bud, how's school going?"

"Okay."

"What are you going to be when you grow up?"

"I don't know," I said tentatively, knowing teenagers were not supposed to have answers to such important questions.

"You know there isn't a better doctor in Ottawa than your father. Your driveway is right next to our bedroom. I don't think a night has gone by when your father hasn't had to go out. You can learn a lot by just watching the way he cares about people."

"I'll think about it," I said as I got up to leave. "Thanks a lot, Uncle Harold."

The next morning I could tell the breakfast atmosphere had changed. The look on Dad's face was an absolute shock to me! He had tears in his eyes. I didn't know what to think.

"Uncle Harold died last night. He had a heart attack. There was nothing I could do."

When I had been in the first grade, I made a sign and hung it on my bedroom door: "DR. BUD GOLLIER — GENERAL PRACTICE." I never seriously considered doing anything else. Relief and excitement were the most prominent emotions in the Gollier household when the mailman delivered my acceptance to the University of Kansas School of Medicine after graduation from college. The excitement was shared by Dad and me. Mother was relieved she wouldn't have to live with two disappointed men.

The curriculum in medical school was well conceived to produce young physicians. The long hours of study afforded many opportunities to realize what it would mean to be called Doctor. Discipline and sacrifice were characteristics that a medical student could not be without. More than anything, all teachers in our classes encouraged each of us to learn to use our minds. We were going to have to learn to be detectives and come up with the right answer.

Pathology class lectures served to initiate medical students to the breadth of knowledge that would be required.

An excellent medical staff of lecturers presented volumes of information about the anatomy of disease. It was nearly impossible to listen to the lecture, watch the slides and take notes at the same time.

Frustration reached its highest point with Dr. Frank "Machine-gun" Mantz at the podium. His rapid-fire delivery of factual information reminded all students of the staccato burst of a machine-gun. Just as I had written down the second word of Dr. Mantz's statement, he would bark, "Next slide," to the projectionist.

Dr. Mantz was an energetic, intent physician who plainly enjoyed his work. He was enthusiastic and reminded me of a Marine sergeant who led his platoon eagerly back up Pork Chop Hill. Dr. Mantz was considerate enough to realize no conscientious student could take notes from his lectures and passed out copies of the notes from which he spoke.

Dr. Mantz was a short, bright-eyed man with the chalky residue of antacid around his mouth and nicotine-tipped fingers. He had a habit of rising to the tips of his toes as he recited the critical point that he did not want forgotten. These were the outward signs of his heightened energy level.

The key to making the proper diagnosis is to be a good observer. It is important to sense what questions to ask, but it is critical to listen to the response. Physical diagnosis lectures were given by Dr. Mahlon Delp to medical school students beginning their clinical years. After two grueling years of basic science studies, these lectures provided the foundation for successful investigation and proper diagnosis for medical students at the University of Kansas.

Dr. Delp began his first lecture by stating there were only three principles in the practice of medicine and we were never to forget them. They were: One — Care of the patient; Two — Care of the patient; and Three — Care of the patient.

The basic science years amounted to long hours of the study and dedication to forming a good basic fund of information. The standing joke was that the textbook of pathology weighed the same as an M-1 rifle. If you didn't learn the course material, you were in great shape for your next career — the Army.

Dr. Delp's physical diagnosis class was my first exposure to applied sciences, an opportunity to apply the accumulated knowledge to problem-solving. Dr. Delp was an expert at "bagging" medical students. He delighted in asking an unsuspecting student a question that stimulated him to learn how to think a problem through. There was always a lot of weight-shifting, hands in pockets and the hem-hawing when "The Silver Fox" was doing the questioning. His piercing eyes, flanking a hawk-like beak, peered out from beneath close-cropped gray hair and bushy eyebrows. His appearance accounted for his nickname, along with a sense that medical students were his natural prey.

One day in Dr. Delp's medical outpatient clinic in my second year, I was taking a history from a 21-year-old boy whose doctor had requested Dr. Delp's consultation because of his reputation as a keen diagnostician. The young man had seen several doctors in central Missouri, and none had been able to diagnose the cause of his dysentery.

"He's lost 30 pounds," his mother said.

The young man was obviously nervous as I took his history and said he had had blood tests and X-rays at two different hospitals and was having diarrhea stools three-four times a day. His physical examination was unremarkable, and there was no abnormality on examination of the abdomen or rectum. I reviewed his tests and they were normal as he had said. As I was preparing my notes to present his case to Dr. Delp, I looked at him again. His eyes were very prominent, and I asked his mother if she had noticed any difference in his eyes.

"No," she said.

"Do you have a picture of him from several years ago?" I asked.

"I have his high school senior picture. It is four years old."

She got it out of her purse and said, "Oh my, his eyes are different!"

He had the prominent eyes of Graves' disease, the exophthalmos due to hyperthyroidism. I re-examined his thyroid gland, paying a little more attention this time and noted it was twice the normal size.

Dr. Delp came in and I presented the case to him and the other students. After the history, I presented the physical findings. I then asked the mother for the picture.

Dr. Delp smiled and punched me in the breastbone with his index finger. He then chuckled and said, "Goddamn it, Gollier, now you're learning to think!"

Then Dr. Delp demonstrated all of the physical findings of hyperthyroidism, the tremor, the rapid pulse, the increased reflexes, the lid lag. It was apparent the young man's sweating had not been due to nerves.

Dr. Delp recommended radioactive iodine therapy. Six months after his treatment, the young man sent me a letter. He said his diarrhea was gone, he had gained 20 pounds and he felt great. His thank you reflected the most meaningful reward in practicing medicine.

The psychiatry service at the Kansas City Veteran's Administration Hospital provided an ideal setting for medical students to study the interaction of patients with thought disorders. The patient population included chronic long-term patients as well as acute cases. When I arrived on the service, I was given a list of five patients I would study and follow during my six-week rotation. The frustration and hopelessness felt by many of the patients were apparent to me as I reviewed the progress notes on my first patient. There were two notes on the last page, both by medical students six weeks apart. As I leafed back through the chart to get a feel for the progress of the patient, I was shocked by the short note as an afterthought on the admission note — Pearl Harbor was bombed yesterday — the date 12-8-41. He had been there more than 20 years! Many long-term patients had learned to master the system. If the social worker or V.A representative started talking about home or rehabilitation, they suddenly started seeing things or threatening people. They were very comfortable in their world. They had no dreams, no family, no goals, and there was no life for them outside the walls of the "Linwood Hilton," our pet name for the V.A. since it was located on Linwood Boulevard.

The new patients usually had an acute problem unless it was a re-admission. We were assigned new patients on a rotating basis. My first new admission was a young man from the boot heel region of southeast Missouri. The challenge with him was that he wouldn't talk. He just sat on the bed and stared at the floor. The most I could get out of him was a grunt. As I looked at the admission note, I learned his name, age and address and could tell he had served in Korea and Japan, and had been medically discharged at Fort Ord in California. He affirmed all the information with grunts. I tried everything I could think of to make him talk. I asked every question that came to mind! Finally I tried the silent treatment. After 10 minutes I noted I was the one getting uneasy, so I left. His physical examination was normal, and his blood chemistries were in the normal range.

I went back the next day and still no response. He would go to the mess hall for meals, but the other patients couldn't get anything out of him either. After three or four days, I was losing my patience. I finally went into his room and pulled a chair up next to his bed. I sat there for about five minutes, then I quietly said, "You're just faking, aren't you? You're afraid to face the world. You're a quitter. What are you running away from? You're just freeloading!"

He startled me as he jumped up and yelled at me, "Sharks! You son-of-a-bitch! That's what I'm running away from! Now are you happy?" Then it all came out.

"I was wounded by a grenade in Korea. After hospitalization in Japan I was to be shipped back to the states for reassignment. As the plane took off I got sick and went to the bathroom at the rear of the plane. Suddenly there was a severe jolt. I was thrown out of the bathroom and smoke and fire was everywhere! I staggered up; it was freezing cold. There was snow on the ground. I looked around and saw the tail section of the airplane. There was fire farther up the slope. A soldier came up to me and asked what unit was I with. When I told him I was on the plane he said, 'That's impossible, everybody is dead!' Later I realized the plane had crashed into Mount Fuji shortly after take-off and 47 GI's on the way home died. I was the only survivor.

"I was reassigned to Fort Ord. When two commercial airliners collided over the Grand Canyon, my unit was called to recover the bodies. As they were lifting the bodies out by helicopter, the chopper I was riding in crashed, killing the two crewmen. I walked away.

"I requested transfer to my old unit in Korea. Then, after transfer, I was a member of the crew of a Navy cargo plane that went down in the Sea of Japan. There were four survivors from the crash. We were floating in the choppy sea in our lifejackets when the sharks came! They hit the radioman first, a young seaman from Georgia. The pilot then saw a floating crate; he told us to climb aboard, but the sharks grabbed the leg of the co-pilot as he scrambled for safety. The pilot and I climbed on the crate. As darkness fell we knew we were in for a long night. The storm blew on and the sharks continued to mill around like guests at a pot-luck banquet waiting for dinner to be served. The crate was losing its buoyancy, the pilot said, "One of us will have to take his chances or neither of us will survive."

Tears started welling in his eyes as he recalled the horror.

"I told him I'd go — he had a family back home and I was single at the time. He told me he was the ranking officer and gave me an order to stay on the crate. He then slipped into the sea and the sharks got him!"

He breathed a sigh of relief and sobbed, "I'm going to lose my job. I've been drinking a quart of vodka a day. My wife wants to leave me and go home to Korea."

I suppressed the urge to suggest he wasn't drinking enough whiskey. We got him into therapy, and with the help of the staff psychiatrist he slowly began to put his life back into order. His wife came and joined him in family counseling. At the end of my rotation, he was making plans to return home. His employer had agreed to reinstate him in his job. His wife was showing some understanding and had agreed to stay with him. That experience taught me that success is often measured by how well we respond to our misfortunes. He was making effective progress in starting a new life and seemed to be putting his horrible memories behind him. My friend from the boot heel of Missouri was going to be a survivor.

Two years later, while at a medical meeting at the university, I saw the staff psychiatrist who had cared for the young man. He told me he was doing fine, working every day and he and his wife had two children.

Finally, I received my medical degree.

As I walked up to my father with my diploma, he smiled and said, "You're real smart now, Buster; you've had a lot of book learning. The most important thing for you to know is what you don't know. Don't ever forget that, son, and never be too proud to admit you can't know everything."

While in medical school, I started dating a school teacher, Mary Lynn Cooper, whom I had known in college. I had not known her well, but I had admired her from a distance. She had been a cheerleader and had dated one of my fraternity brothers. I should have sensed something special was in store for me when she agreed to pick me up at 5 a.m. at the Kansas City Veterans' Hospital for our first date. I had been on call all night, and we were going to Columbia, Missouri, to watch the Kansas-Missouri football game. She got a taste of the life of a physician's wife when I was delayed two hours by an emergency. She was unperturbed by the delay, and we were off to a great start! The Kansas loss didn't discourage either of us, and we were married a year later during my senior year of medical school.

During our courtship, my parents had invited us to spend a weekend with them at Bull Shoals Lake in Arkansas for some crappie fishing. Dad had arranged a guide for Mary Lynn and me, as he felt that would ensure I had an opportunity to fish as well. Mary Lynn had no problem throwing the small jig on an ultra-light rod we had rigged for her.

As we left the dock the first morning, the frost was in the air as the sun slowly rose in the east. Large flocks of mallards were passing through on their way north and there was a lot of activity. The dogwoods were in bloom and we had a lot of fun enjoying the sights and each other.

Suddenly Mary Lynn screamed, "I've got one!" and she pulled in a plump two-pound crappie.

"How deep are you fishing?" asked Grey Richardson, our guide, who had a pig farm near Tucker Hollow a few miles away.

Mary Lynn looked at him blankly, "How would I know?"

A few minutes later she had another and then another and another. Each time Grey put a fish on the stringer she would look blankly at him when he tried to get an idea as to the depth of the crappie. As he unhooked her sixth crappie before either of us had a strike, he looked at her sternly, "Young lady, this may be your last fishing trip!"

Things couldn't have been better. We were married the next year. After interning in another part of the country, we returned to a nearby city to serve a year of internal medicine residency at Metropolitan Hospital where my father interned and my mother received her nurse's training.

I had been very fortunate to be accepted as a resident at Metropolitan, where I had done histories and physicals as an extern during the summers of medical school when I hadn't been a guide at Great Bear Lake. My father knew many of the staff physicians and referred many of his patients to Metro. Mother also had a lot of friends from her nurse's training days. The staff doctors were all committed to education and were inspiring teachers.

My favorite was Dr. Matthew Drake. He was a droll, no-nonsense man who was a keen diagnostician. He had a distinct cock to his head, and his shuffling gait and mild tremor when he wrote belied his early Parkinson's disease. It did not take him long to get the critical part of a patient's history. After examining the patient, the residents and interns would gather around him, and he would efficiently dissect the case and recover "the pearls" of information that he felt were useful for teaching purposes. Time was never a major concern on rounds. The main priority was to learn.

One day Dr. Drake was discussing the tenaciousness required to solve a perplexing problem.

"You have to take advantage of all your resources. You must use your eyes and ears and think logically. Don't forget to use the eyes and ears of the nurses. Take the time to listen to them. Practicing good medicine requires teamwork.

I reminded Dr. Drake that although we were a generation apart, we both had our intellectual curiosity inspired in the same environment. We had lived in the same fraternity which had diligently lived up to its motto — The Pursuit of Excellence. To strive for the highest standards was a goal that had been bred into each of us separately during our undergraduate days.

I remember one day during a discussion of the adrenal gland and its function, Dr. Drake said, "You've got to learn to think teleologically. There's a reason for everything." The reason the blood cortisol is twice as high in the morning as in the evening is to help the fox chase the hare. He needs his eyes to be sharp and dilated in the early morning hours to help in the restricted light, and he needs the energy and faster heart rate with improved reflexes to chase and catch the hare."

He was also an expert on the evaluation of low sodium, which can cause mental changes that can mimic circulation problems. He floored me one day when he asked me to explain Inappropriate ADH Secretion.

"What did you say?" I stammered.

He repeated himself and asked me to look it up for a report the next day. That was when I first learned about a clinical condition that is terribly common and relatively easy to treat when recognized. Fluid restriction is unbelievably effective and a relatively simple blood and urine test will confirm the diagnosis. The ironic thing about this condition is that replacing the sodium deficiency simply makes the problem worse and increased sodium excretion by the kidneys. It was my dream to learn to be as perceptive as Dr. Drake. His enthusiasm for teaching was infectious and he made the practice of medicine more enjoyable.

The only problem in practicing medicine was an interruption of my residency by a call to Vietnam.

Near the end of my residency, Mary Lynn and I were watching television one evening when President Lyndon Johnson addressed the nation and stated he would not be a candidate for re-election in 1968.

"However, I will not be a lame duck president," he told the nation. In his commitment to resolve the stalemate in Vietnam, he committed an additional 65,000 U.S. Army troops to the war effort. A chill crept over me as I sensed the impact of that decision on my military obligation. I had an Air Force Commission and was awaiting active duty orders. My fears were well founded as I received a letter from the Department of Air Force one week later. The letter began:

"Dear Captain Gollier:

As a result of a change in military man-power allocations, the Air Force now has more physicians than is required to meet its needs. As a result your commission has been transferred to the U.S. Army. The transfers were selected by lot. That's the way the ball bounces."

"At least they didn't say that's the way the cookie crumbles," I said to Mary Lynn, trying unsuccessfully to brighten her up.

In a short time, my orders to Vietnam arrived.

At the year-end banquet at Metropolitan Hospital, all the residents were asked to reveal their plans for practice and future training. When my turn came, I said softly, "I have a one-year sabbatical in trauma and tropical disease in the Republic of Vietnam."

The news was not all bad that spring, as we also learned Mary Lynn was pregnant with expected delivery of our first child in January, halfway through our year of separation.

EIGHT

I ARRIVED at the Bien Hoa Air Base near Saigon in the middle of an October night in 1968. It was hot and humid. We were taken to a tent and given our unit assignments. As I walked to the bunkhouse after receiving my assignment, I passed a large bunker. Written on the front of the bunker in bold black print was the message: "A pessimist is a man who sleeps in his body bag."

I was assigned to an artillery battalion that was located near Saigon, and I settled into the role of Army doctor.

The choice was bright heat and dark heat. I chose the canvas shade of the battalion-aid station. It was hot, but it was quiet. I took my shirt off, lay down on the cot and turned on the fan. I noted the ubiquitous staccato "chop-chop" of the helicopter cutting its way through the heat in the background. This one was coming my way, making another delivery to the grave-registration battalion across the road. I watched them unload their cargo one time. They had 18 young marines who had been ambushed in the Delta. The bodies were distorted by blast and fire beyond recognition. Identification was the only task remaining before embalming and preparation for the final flight home. My hand went to my neck absent-mindedly. I grasped my dog tags on the crude chain around my neck. "Better there than on my toe," I thought, and decided once was enough to watch them unload their cargo. The sign at their gate said it all: COMPANY B (MED)735th SUPPORT BATTALION (MORTUARY) "WELCOME TO HARD TIMES."

The mosquitoes weren't even moving around. They were all clinging to the undersides of the canvas. I didn't bother to swat at them. I turned on the radio. The Armed Forces Radio Network was carrying the World Series. Bob Gibson of the Cardinals vs. Denny McClain of the Tigers. I was a Cardinal fan. I opened a can of Budweiser to cheer them on.

A broad hulk darkened the doorway of my tent.

"Captain Gollier?" a voice said.

"Come in." I turned down the radio.

"I'm Sergeant Houleran, sir." He had a friendly face.

His short haircut was typical military — all regulation. The handlebar mustache was his way of saying he was his own man.

I offered him a beer as I noted his Special Forces insignia.

"No thanks, sir. I'm the medic with the Special Forces out in the province. We serve as advisors to the South Vietnamese. The wife of the village chief in my area had a baby several weeks ago. She's running a temperature and has some foul-smelling drainage."

"How's the baby?" I asked.

"Seems fine. We're feeding her goat's milk. I didn't think she should nurse with the chills and fever."

"Who delivered the baby?"

"I did." He seemed almost upset that I had asked. "She had an easy delivery. I didn't even have to cut her."

"That was my next question. How long did she flow after delivery?"

"About a week. Lots of clots at first, then bad cramps. Finally the cramps quit and the bleeding stopped."

"Sounds like she's got endometritis. Probably a gram-negative bacterial infection. She needs to go to the hospital."

"I know, but she won't go."

"Why not?"

"She doesn't trust Vietnamese doctors."

"That's a hellava note."

"Will you help me?"

"How can I help you?"

"Come with me and tell me what to do."

"I've already told you."

"I know, sir, but her husband, the village chief, won't let me take her to the hospital either. He wants an American doctor."

"Well, I'll have to ask my C.O."

"He's already said yes."

I felt like I had been set up. "You've already cleared it?"

"Yes, sir."

"Let's get started. How far?"

"About 15 kilometers. We have to walk through a rice paddie the last two kliks. It's even footing, but knee deep. If you stay right behind me, you'll be fine."

"If you stop suddenly, you'll find out I follow orders."

The rainy season had just ended and the roads were all mud with water standing in puddles all along the way.

I laughed to myself at the contradictions I offered, a medical bag in my left hand and a .45 on my right hip.

After about an hour, Houleran stopped the jeep. "We walk from here."

The walk wasn't as bad as I feared. We waded along a road beside the rice paddy. The village was nestled at the edge of a dense tropical forest. There were 10 or 12 grass shelters visible as the road curved to our left.

"How big is the village?" I asked.

"There are about 30 hooches. I don't know how many people. The men are in the Army. Only the wives and kids are here. The bigger hooch is where we'll find Mama-san." He walked over and yelled something I couldn't understand. A small Vietnamese man came out and looked at me. He waved, smiled broadly, revealing teeth that had seen better days and offered his hand.

"Thank you. Thank you," he smiled and nodded eagerly. Houleran motioned me to the doorway of the hooch.

"Let's meet the patient." I ducked and followed him into the darkness. There were two steps. The packed clay floor was covered with a bamboo rug. There was a low bed in the far corner. A young face peered at me from beneath some covers. Houleran said something. The only word I recognized was Collier. Close enough, I thought, as I bowed in acknowledging the introductions.

I felt her forehead. She had a fever, but not high. Her pulse was fast at 110. Her blood pressure was 110/60. I placed the blood-pressure cuff and stethoscope back in the bag and found a light. Her ears and throat were normal. Her abdomen was only mildly tender. I picked up the light again and told Houleran to ask her to stick out her tongue. He didn't ask.

He showed her what to do. She giggled softly and stuck out her tongue. No evidence of dehydration — a good sign.

"Is she taking fluid well?"

He nodded yes.

"Now for the tough part, the pelvic exam."

"We're going to need better light," I said to Houleran.

"We could reflect light from a Coleman lantern off the mirror I use to shave."

"Now you're thinking. What about a vaginal speculum?"

"I have one. I got it at the field hospital in Saigon."

"You mean they gave it to you?"

"You might say that. You learn to be resourceful in the Special Forces."

I asked Houleran to explain the procedure to the young woman. She seemed to trust Houleran. I was beginning to trust him, too. We set up the lantern and mirror. I got down on my knees. We adjusted the light and moved the young woman to the edge of the bed. The bed was constructed of bamboo. I told Houleran to ask her to place her feet together and spread her knees. I could see a thick bloody discharge, not necessarily unusual at two weeks postpartum. I inserted the speculum and inspected the vagina. No evidence of any tears. The cervix was easily visible. Houleran's lighting system was quite effective. There was a moderate amount of bloody discharge from the cervix. I took a swab and placed it in a culture tube. I removed the speculum, carefully spread the labia with the fingers of my gloved hand. I asked Houleran to ask her to relax. He tried, but she was still tense. I told Houleran to call for her husband.

"He won't come in. He says he doesn't have the stomach for this."

Houleran smiled at the young woman and patted her on the shoulder.

I needed to assess the size of her uterus and evaluate whether any infection was present in the ovaries or tubes. Slowly she seemed to relax. I was able to move the cervix. It was a little tender, but not bad. The uterus was enlarged, but not soft or boggy. There was no other mass in the pelvis.

"She either has endometritis or a urinary tract infection,"

I said to Houleran.

"We'll get a culture of the cervical discharge, and we need a urine specimen for a culture. I'll draw some blood for a culture, a blood count and creatinine. We can take the samples by the field hospital on our way home. They'll be our laboratory, Houleran."

"Doc, you think they'll do it for you?"

"No, I think they'll do it for you. You're the resourceful one. Now, let's get on our way."

I bid the patient and her husband farewell and off we went.

"What's the creatinine for, sir?" asked Houleran as we walked back to the Jeep.

"You asked me to tell you what to do. We're going to try one more time to talk her husband into letting us take her to the Province Hospital. The field hospital can't take civilians. If they refuse, we'll have to start antibiotics while we're waiting for the culture. If she doesn't have allergies, we can give her Ampicillin capsules by mouth. But to cover the most likely bacteria, we'll need another drug. Gentamicin would give us broader coverage, but it can cause kidney damage. The blood creatinine level is a measure of the renal function. It will help us determine the right dose for her weight."

The lab tech at the Field Hospital was very helpful. I presented the samples, complete with requisitions, identifying the patient as Corporal Willie Daniels of the 23rd Artillery Group. I described the sample from the cervix as taken from the left eye. I included Daniel's SSN and MOS. There were no questions asked.

I requisitioned some Ampicillin and Gentamicin from the pharmacy and instructed Houleran to give our patient 250 mg. of Ampicillin four times a day orally and 35 mg. of Gentamicin intramuscularly every eight hours.

"A shot?" he asked in disbelief.

"It's the only way to given Gentamicin. Sorry for the trouble."

"Okay, sir."

"Take her temperature twice a day and be sure she drinks at least a four-ounce glass of liquid every hour. Report to me by radio every day and come get me every other day and I'll make a hooch call."

"Yes, sir." Houleran reported as instructed and I called on the patient every other day for 10 days. On the fifth day, I stopped by the lab to check on the cultures. The lab tech gave me a strange look. "That Daniels has a weird infection in his eye. You'd better get him on an antibiotic. We grew out a gram-negative rod. It's sensitive to Ampicillin and Gentamicin, but it was a heavy growth. That bug is usually only seen in the urinary tract."

"He's a strange young man," I called out as I left.

"Thanks a lot."

Houleran was waiting in the Jeep. I hopped in and said, "Let's go see our patient."

"How were the tests, sir?"

"Okay."

"What are you smiling about?"

"Nothing. Was I smiling?"

"You look like the cat that ate the canary."

"I was just thinking that there is a little humor in everything if you look hard enough."

"What's funny about this?"

"It seems Corporal Willie Daniels has really been eyeing the women."

Houleran chuckled. "I wondered how you got them to do those tests. You can be resourceful, too."

"We need to draw some blood for another creatinine and white blood count today. We found out the Ampicillin and Gentamicin will be effective. Only five more days of the antibiotics."

When we got to the village, we were delighted to see our patient, her husband and infant daughter all sitting in front of their hooch. They were all smiles and waved as we approached. I checked her abdomen and drew a blood sample. As I prepared to leave, they brought out a bottle and four glasses. They both took one and gave one to Houleran and me.

"Rice wine," said Houleran. "He makes it himself. Not bad, either."

Wine was poured for all. We all had seconds. Houleran was talking with them in what I took as Vietnamese. Finally, the chief and his wife looked at me, raised their glasses and said, "USA Number one," and gave me a big smile. I shook their hands and said, "You, number one, too."

The battalion received orders to move to the city of Tay Ninh, Tay Ninh Province, 12 to 15 kilometers from Cambodia. I was told that here was a convoy leaving for Tay Ninh the next morning and I was to ride with the convoy. The convoy was referred to as "The Orient Express." It was a 120-kilometer ride over dusty roads through the heart of the rice paddies and rubber plantations, which had served as the staging area for most of the combat in the bloody Tet Offensive that occurred one year previously when the Communists had attacked Saigon directly. The Orient Express had a history of being ambushed several times every month as it supplied many of the army units in the area near the Cambodian border.

On our way to Tay Ninh, we passed through the Michelin rubber plantation near Cu Chi. It was beautiful. The groves of rubber trees were undisturbed and seemed out of place in a country so scarred by war.

"The rubber trees seem immune to the defoliant spray that has affected the jungle all around," I said.

"That's one of the strange rules we have to play in this war," said Major Maguffin, a salty regular army officer who was beginning his second tour of duty in Vietnam. "The rubber is one of their big cash crops and is a major export product. We have to pay $75 to the Saigon government for every rubber tree damaged or destroyed. Therefore, the Michelin plantation is off-limits to B-52 strikes and defoliants. This is where the Tet Offensive originated. Guess where the Viet Cong stronghold is? It's hell for our boys to get hit and have their buddies killed and not be able to chase the V.C. into this damned haven of theirs!"

Bull sessions with my fellow officers gave me insight into military strategy and I was involved in staff meetings in a peripheral manner. My part was limited to a brief report of illness and injuries and a report of latrine inspections. I was compelled to follow occasionally to inspect damage after a mortar attack. One evening two mortar rounds came in and the damage directly involved me as the mortar rounds had flattened two of the three latrines I had just inspected prior to the attack. One of my closest friends was Captain Warren "Deuce" Johnson, a West Point graduate, who was our S-2 or intelligence officer. Deuce and his non-commissioned officer, Sergeant John Thiery, a ruddy-faced, happy-go-lucky man from San Francisco, would go out to perform a "Shell rep." By inspecting the impact area, they could calculate the back-azimuth, or the direction from which the round had come. Then after digging out the shell fragments and determining the type of round, one could pinpoint its site of origin by knowing the range of the ordnance. Deuce would call the artillery battery and they would blanket the area with some well-placed "friendly fire."

"One of these days they're going to figure you out, Deuce," I said to Warren one evening as he phoned in the map reading to the artillery gunner. "The V.C are gonna put another round in the same tube five minutes after the first and we're all gonna buy the farm!"

"You worry too much, Doc. They're always on the move. They wouldn't think of that."

"Don't be too sure."

Sick call in the aid station was primarily restricted to skin rashes, venereal disease and evaluation of general complaints that often were due to malingering. In order to combat boredom, our unit participated in a medical civic action program and provided medical care for several small villages in the area. The commanding officer told me I would have to arrange for our own security, so I insisted my medics and I be issued M-16's. He reluctantly agreed and we were able to encourage other GIs to accompany us when they had a day off, and they provided cover while they were taking pictures of the villages to send home. We never had any difficulty and didn't see the enemy, or didn't recognize the enemy. We provided care for about 500 Vietnamese each week. I was surprised that there were so many young men loitering around in one village we attended. I would see 20 to 30 of them every day we held clinic there. I wondered why they weren't in the army. After I left the country, one of my fellow officers wrote and told me they *were* in the army — the other army. The North Vietnamese, Sixth Division had been tunneled in under the village, and they had been routed out by the infantry in a fire fight. I shuddered as I read his letter and realized how lucky I had been they hadn't decided to transfer my commission to their unit.

One night after going to my bunk, I heard the staccato burst of M-16 rifle fire on our perimeter. There were screams of "Doc, Doc, come quick!" I went to the guard post and saw a young GI riddled across the chest with bullet wounds. As I pronounced him dead, I heard a sob coming from the bunker. A young soldier was telling the MP, "I thought he was a V.C. Johnny was my best friend!" As I sat down beside them, I saw the smoldering joint in the corner. I picked it up and confirmed my suspicion — marijuana.

One day I hopped the command chopper on a run to An Loc just 40 kilometers north of us. We had a firing battery there, and I needed to make a routine inspection. A medical school classmate, Ernie Neighbor, was assigned to a provincial hospital there, and I decided to pay him a visit.

Ernie greeted me with a smile as I stepped off the helicopter.

"We never get hit. It's peaceful as can be. I live in a nice French villa and have a lot of free time."

Thirty minutes after I arrived, the mortars started coming in. The second one hit the top of a palm tree adjacent to the villa. I met Ernie in the bunker. He was dressed in his shorts, cowboy boots, helmet and a flak jacket.

"Thanks for coming, Bud," he said, only half smiling. "There are some casualties over at the hospital halfway across town. Why don't you come along? At least you've got a M-16."

"Might as well. It sure is peaceful here."

We hopped into Ernie's Jeep and sped through the dark city. On the way, Ernie turned on the radio. A garbled transmission mentioned an unconfirmed report that K-1, K-2 and K-3 were on a line moving fast toward An Loc.

"What's that mean?" Ernie muttered.

"You don't want to know," I said, remembering that those

were the code names for three North Vietnamese divisions located just 10 kilometers away, across the Cambodian border. We rushed into the hospital. Ernie attended the casualty, a small child with minor wounds, while I went back to the radio. There was no further mention of the imminent invasion that my mind was prepared for. When Ernie came out, an all clear was broadcast. I gave him a full report.

"I hope you'll be leaving on the first chopper out in the morning, good friend. You sure know how to fuck up a good deal. That's the first time we've been hit in six months."

The Vietnam experience was not one that provided strength of character, but the separation from family helped put my priorities in order. As my year neared its end, I was summoned to headquarters to fill out my request for assignment to the states. Vietnam veterans were given first choice of state side assignments. The personnel officer, a lieutenant, asked me what my first choice was.

"Fort Riley."

"Fort Riley?" he asked, startled. "In Kansas? No one ever asks for Fort Riley. Why in the world would you ask for Fort Riley?"

"It's close to home."

There was a brief going-away party for Sergeant Thiery and me as we were scheduled to leave for home on the same plane two days later. Early the next morning, the commanding officer notified me that there was space on a "freedom bird," our term for flights home. That morning I was already packed, so a medic took me to the airport and I was on my way a day early.

The flight home was accompanied by heightened anticipation. The long year was over. The detour in my training had been successfully breached. I was soon to be reunited with family and meet my son.

Mary Lynn, Mom, Dad, Fred, Mary Lynn's parents and a score of friends from home were wildly waving at the gate as I walked down the steps off the jet at the Kansas City Airport. Mary Lynn had her arms full of a bright-eyed child who didn't seem afraid of me as she thrust him into my arms. Bo was seven months old and seemed to enjoy the celebration.

We proceeded to Ottawa, and Dad charbroiled steaks for all.

After I returned home, I sent a few letters to Deuce. After several months, I finally got a reply. The return address was Camp Zama, Japan.

Dear Doc,

Well, you were right. The night after you left, we had a mortar attack. Sgt. Thiery and I went out to take a shell rep. While we were digging, another round came in. Sgt. Thiery was killed. I received a leg wound and I am now hospitalized in Japan. As you know, Sgt. Thiery was leaving the next day. His tour of duty was over. I told him to stay in the barracks, but you know how hard-working he was. He planned to be back home in San Francisco for the Giants' opener.

Hope to see you in the States sometime.

Your friend,
Deuce

NINE

WE MADE FREQUENT TRIPS to Ottawa from Fort Riley, and with only a little prompting, Bo took to calling Dad, "Big Daddy." Mom was quick to say, "I will not be Big Mama!"

Mary Lynn said, "How about Big Nelle?"

"That's not so bad."

So Big Daddy and Big Nelle they became.

After the year at Fort Riley, it was time to settle down. Mary Lynn and I agreed to raise our family in my hometown, and I joined my father and his partner, Dr. David Laury, in practice. We had a thriving family practice, and my family enjoyed the contented life we shared.

Mary Lynn remembers it like this:

. . . . Yes, we had a very comfortable life, but I was very apprehensive when we first moved back to Bud's hometown. When we were dating, we would come for dinner to see Bud's folks. As we got out of the city into the countryside, Bud would say, "I can smell it — God's country. We're getting closer." When I accepted his proposal of marriage, I knew also that I had accepted his plan to live in his hometown and to go into practice with his father.

I was an only child and had grown up in a big city. I wasn't sure I would adapt to the small-town life. I thought that the small town would be a fine place to raise a family. We bought an older home in an older neighborhood of the community, and I was really excited when we first agreed to move into our new home! However, it needed a lot of work, and I really became involved in the planning stages in many home improvements. The kitchen needed to be redone; we needed a new roof; and since our lifestyle was oriented to the outdoors, we planned a new patio and did some land-scaping.

Our anxiety about being childless had been termi-nated by Bo's birth four months after Bud left for Viet-nam. I missed him terribly during labor and even more as I was holding our son after delivery. I was then very eager to be a part of a family community.

When Bud returned from Vietnam, I knew he was eager to meet his son, but also more excited than ever to return to the familiar good things he had remem-bered as a youth. We were stationed at a nearby army base for a year prior to setting up practice. It was ex-citing to spend weekends looking for our dream house, and I was somewhat apprehensive to move into a 50-year-old-English Tudor home. After we moved in, we soon found that John was on the way, and we quickly began to fill up the space along with a bouncing Irish Setter puppy Bud received from one of his father's pa-tients as soon as we moved in.

A year later, our family was complete as Sara Jane arrived. She had my mother's red hair and was named after her Aunt Jane, Bud's sister, who had passed away from Hodgkin's disease the year before we were married.

We loved our family home and the friendly com-munity that was to be our haven forever.

The fall was an enchanting time as our tree-lined streets were bordered by majestic maples and elms, and the brick street lent a quaint aura to the neighborhood. It was particularly exciting during the fall afternoons when the junior high band marched down our street and all the neighborhood children donned their par-ents' New Year's Eve hats and marched along with the band.

We were close to several reservoirs, which gave us the opportunity to enjoy water activities, and it was particularly fun to have the opportunity to learn about such endeavors as mushroom hunting, quail hunting and ice skating, which I had never had an opportunity to appreciate as a child. The children really enjoyed the opportunity to make new friends and to share experiences with them.

Our church life was particularly rewarding, and both Bud and I enjoyed immensely the experiences our children had at their Sunday school. It was particularly rewarding when all three children, one Sunday morning in church, decided to go forward and ask for baptism in front of the congregation. It was a complete surprise to both of us as they made that decision on their own. . . .

Just as Mom and Dad had been committed to family vacations during my youth, Mary Lynn and I decided that would be a priority of ours. We had enjoyed snow skiing from our college days, and we both loved the scenic Rocky Mountains in the winter. The thin air, coupled with vigorous exercise, was refreshing to us both, and we started the children out on skis the first winter after they could walk. They all took to it eagerly and by their second ski trip they could ski with Mary Lynn and me, and it was all we could do to keep up with them.

I was determined to learn as much as I could from my father as I started practicing medicine. He had started out during the late 1930s, when the depression was still fresh in everybody's mind.

"Office calls were $1.50 or whatever the patient could pay," he would say.

I remember someone was always at the back door with a dozen eggs, a couple of chickens, a bag of roasting ears, green beans or squash. I would say, "Thank you very much."

"Tell your Dad it's from the Johnsons."

It was many years later that I realized most of those people were paying on a baby or an appendectomy, and in their own way the patient was satisfying his account.

By 1970, I had a good education, both in the classroom and in the bunkers and hamlets of Vietnam, and my studies as well as my experience with summer jobs had instilled the work ethic in me.

After Mary Lynn and I moved to Ottawa, we were having

dinner one evening with Dad and Mom. After dinner, Dad and I moved to the living room. Diagnosis and treatment of various illnesses were not the things that worried me. I was more interested in learning the art of medicine from my father.

"Dad, tell me some of the things I need to know about setting up practice."

"A few of the things I am going to tell you are things they don't teach in medical school.

"The first thing you need to do is get an early start. Have your day organized so you can always respond to an emergency. I believe in making early rounds so I don't have any surprises before I get to the office. And you must always be available. You and Dave will be alternating calls, but you must be willing to respond even if you aren't on call. If you always respond to the telephone, the patient will get the impression that their welfare is your first priority. You can always tell them that your partner is on call, but since you know the particulars of the case, you may be more comfortable responding yourself. That attitude will pay big dividends in the future. That is the primary reason my patients have been so loyal since I semi-retired after my heart attack. Always give the patient your time — that's all you have to sell. Look the patient in the eye. Make them think they are the only patient you have. If you get too busy to take care of people, they will get the message and go somewhere else. There are a couple of other things to remember. I have never changed medicine just for the sake of change. When you send a patient to a specialist, he will usually make some change, however insignificant, to justify his fee. I remember one time I saw a patient, and he asked if I minded if he got a second opinion. I arranged for him to go to the city to see a specialist. Before he left, he asked me to list his diagnoses, which I did. Six weeks later he came back, mad as hell, and said, 'I was in the hospital five days and when I left, he handed me a list of the same three diagnoses that you had made. It cost me $600.'

" 'Maybe you would have been happier if he had said you had cancer,' I told him.

"Your first obligation is to rule out organic or serious illnesses. The key to being a successful physician is to be certain that when the patient gets well they are on your medicine. Time and patience will cure many maladies after you have eliminated reversible disease. And another thing, always do business with your patients. You may be able to save a few pennies by shopping in the city, but it is important to your patients and your community that you trade locally as often as possible.

"The most important thing for you to learn, Bud, is that nurses are your partners. You should always read the nurses' notes before you make rounds. They do not write in the chart to practice penmanship. Remember, they have been in attendance of the patient 24 hours a day. You need to take advantage of their assessment. They don't make rounds with you just to carry the charts. If you make them feel as if their input is important to you, they will help you in uncountable ways.

"And one more thing. You will not always be right. It is not your duty to be right all the time. It is your duty to always give your best effort and learn from unexpected outcomes."

I had not been in practice too long when I had an opportunity to apply several of my father's principles. The phone rang one morning at 3 o'clock, and the nurse in the emergency room reported a teenage boy had come with his parents, who stated he was having an asthma attack and they wanted him to be given a shot of adrenaline. The patient was just traveling through town on his way home from vacation when they stopped at the emergency room. I told the nurse that I would be there shortly.

"All they want is a shot of adrenaline," was her response.

"I don't know the patient, and if they are sick enough to come to an Emergency Room, they are sick enough to see a doctor. I'll be right out."

As I walked in the emergency room, I noted a teenage boy acutely short of breath, accompanied by his obviously anxious parents — one on each side.

As I laid my stethoscope on his chest, I first noted to my

surprise the absence of the musical wheezing associated with acute asthma. I then became aware of another presence in the room. It first affected my eyes with a sense of burning and then the pungent odor took me back to chemistry lab — acetone.

I quickly looked at the nurse and said, "We have an emergency on our hands! Get me a bottle of intravenous fluid and 100 units of insulin."

It was apparent his shortness of breath was not due to asthma, but rather was the air hunger associated with diabetic ketoacidosis.

I drew blood for the sugar and other baseline chemistries that were required and told the parents he would have to stay in Medical Intensive Care for a few days. The blood test confirmed the diagnosis, but I had already started the intravenous insulin. Three days later his sugars were under control and he was dismissed to continue his journey home.

....

I continued my professional relationship with many of the doctors at Metro. They were always available for telephone consultations, and I had an opportunity to exchange case histories with them at medical meetings. They were also my primary source of referral when I had a complicated problem. My special interest was cardiology, and I felt the patients in our community would benefit if I could learn the technique of implanting a temporary heart pacemaker through the vein when heart rhythm problems occurred during an acute heart attack. The heart specialists at Metro were very cooperative and agreed to sponsor a six-week fellowship to teach me the technique, as well as treatment of other medical complications that can occur in an Intensive Care Unit. It was a very rewarding time, and the supervision and instruction were excellent.

It was not long after I returned home that a patient developed a complete heart block in our hospital. I was anxious as I threaded the pacemaker into the femoral vein. I watched it carefully on the X-ray fluoroscope as it passed through the vena cava and then made the critical turn into the right atrium of the heart and then through the tricuspid valve into the apex of the right ventricle where it could do its pacing. I then hooked the battery pack to the electrodes and watched the monitor — perfect. I was relieved that things had gone without a hitch. Having that capability in our hospital would be a great service and avoid the need to depend on drugs alone while making the emergency ambulance run to a hospital equipped to put in pacemakers.

TEN

MERLE PRICE, a retired car dealer, had long been one of my father's closest friends. Dad, Merle, Cliff Haverty and Jim Frizzell had taught Fred and me the fine points of hunting, fishing, companionship and conservation.

After he retired, Merle became acquainted with a man who shared both his love for fishing and his independence.

George Hary had owned a bait shop in Stover, Missouri. He had a good business with numerous fishing reservoirs in the area. But he found the business too confining to pursue his passion — the North country!

George sold his business and was able to realize his dream of building a cabin in the remote part of the North. After he built his first cabin, he felt he had to build another. He had it down to a science. He would stake out an island or a point for his cabin site and would obtain a 99-year lease from the Canadian government. He felt 99 years was probably long enough, but was certain he would be given an option to renew his lease when the time came. George would arrange for lumber and other materials to be transported to the site by tractor train over the ice in the winter. The next summer he would hire two carpenters and they would fly in and put up the cabin. He would spend a week in the spring and a week in the fall at the cabin for a few years and would sell it to an acquaintance and move on to a different challenge. His cabins were of simple plywood construction, but provided adequate shelter. They were used by trappers and hunters in the desolate winters. The natives treated the cabins very respectfully, hoping for the same shelter during another winter.

George needed a fishing companion, and Merle had both the time and inclination. George built a cabin on the east arm of Great Slave Lake in 1965. The cabin was on a small island near the mainland. George called it Robin Island, after a family of robins who kept him company while he built it. George and Merle made several trips to the cabin on Robin Island. One year Merle could tell George was more irritable than usual. Merle was sipping a cup of coffee when George interrupted his thoughts.

"Merle, we need to make a trip over to my old cabin by Snowdrift to get the propane icebox I stashed back in the bush," George said while clearing the table after breakfast.

"How far is it?" asked Merle.

"About 65 miles! One hundred and thirty round trip."

"It'll take over two hours to get there."

"More like four!"

Merle frowned, thinking how to say he'd rather take a beating than miss a day fishing. "Let the hide go with the hair," he said as he looked wistfully out the back window at the bay behind the cabin.

"What was that?" George said as he poured the last of the coffee down the drain.

"Nothing."

"I'll go down to the boat and gas up. We'd better leave before the wind comes up!"

Merle fumed. Sixty-five miles of bouncing his butt on the hard seat during the boat ride. One hundred thirty miles round trip.

"Heaven save us, Mrs. Davis," he said to himself in the empty cabin as he put on his rain suit to protect him from the spray that was bound to come after the waves picked up in the afternoon. The lake was an old millpond on a breathless day as they left the dock.

Merle was unsettled. It was bad enough that he wanted to be fishing. He didn't trust the weather.

"I'd ask the dealer for a new hand, but we're playing George's game," Merle mused. The attempts to occupy his mind with futile exercises and plots to devise a way of escape provided Merle with an illusion of gallows humor.

Merle looked at his watch again. Then he looked closer to be certain the second hand was moving.

They rounded Et-Then Island. Red Cliff loomed in front of them.

"Not hard to see where it got its name!" George shouted above the din of the 20-horsepower Johnson motor, pointing to the deep red cliffs vividly revealing their rich iron and copper composition. "We're in Christie Bay now. Feel how much cooler it is when the breeze comes off the water rather than the island? I call this the icebox of the world."

Merle forced a smile. He had heard this line ten times. His frown returned.

George was not discouraged. "The wind's coming up a little. The weather report said a front might be moving in from the west."

Merle was discouraged. "If you knew that, why the hell are we making this trip?"

"We need that icebox!"

"Like I need a dose of the clap."

"What was that?" George shouted.

"I didn't say anything."

"We'll be there in a hour and a half. Hope the Indians didn't find that icebox! I had it pretty well hidden."

Merle reached into the sack under the bow and got an apple. He handed one to George.

"This isn't too bad, is it, Merle?"

Merle shrugged.

The lake was a little rougher as they passed Red Cliff and the south wind had a longer stretch to fan the lake.

After 20 minutes of ducking spray and flexing his hamstrings every time he felt the bow release from contact with the lake, Merle sighed as George almost mercifully turned the boat in the direction of the wind. The rhythm of the bouncing was different and the boat settled softly into the swells after generating enough speed to break through the rollers.

"Around the next point, on the right!" George shouted

Merle felt relieved. Maybe he could take a snooze before they headed back. At least he could find his bottle of Crown Royal in the shore lunch box and have a little "nippy."

They rounded the point. The cabin was in poor repair. The two front windows were broken. A tree had fallen against the north side and damaged the roof.

"This cabin is 20 years old. It's too close to the settlement of Snowdrift. The fishing isn't as good here because of all the boats. The natives commercial fish here as well. That's why I moved to the other cabin."

Merle was only half listening while looking for the whiskey in the lunch box.

"I left it in the cabin, Merle," George said, his craggy face breaking into a smile.

Merle hung his head, then moved to the front seat and kneeled as the boat slowly coasted into the flat rock. Merle got out and tied the boat. He turned to offer George a hand. George was grinning. In his hand was a bottle of Crown Royal.

"It's about time for a little chocolate to come into my life," Merle said.

"I'll go get the icebox; then we'll head back."

"I think I'll take a little snooze."

"No, a storm's coming up. If the wind really picks up from the south, we'll never make it across that final 10 miles from Et-Then Island to the cabin."

Merle dipped his cup in the water. The water was so cold he could feel the skin on the back of his hand get taut. The pulsating discomfort was quickly relieved as he raised his cup. He took a drink and his gullet was soothed as the cool, clear water rolled down to his stomach. He poured just enough Crown Royal into the cup to give the drink the appearance of freshly made ice tea.

"Not too much, Merle," George said. "You may need to run the boat back."

Merle knew better. George was always the pilot. He didn't need help. He needed company or an audience.

"I'll go check the icebox."

Merle got his boat cushion and lay down on the moss, using the cushion as a pillow for his head. A big mosquito was on his hand. He slapped him. Then several more were on his wrist. He rubbed his brow and felt several more mosquitoes. He stood up and walked toward the point. There was a breeze there and the mosquitoes might not be as thick. His cup was empty. He knelt down by the flat rocks next to the boat and filled his cup again. Another shot of Crown Royal. He took a drink and let its warmth settle in the pit of his stomach.

"This isn't so bad," he thought.

George's shout brought him back to his senses.

"Come give me a hand, Merle! The icebox is right where I left it. I could carry it, but the ground is so rocky I'm not sure of my footing. Two of us could handle it better."

"Or have twice as much trouble with the footing," Merle mumbled.

"What was that?"

"I didn't say anything."

They picked up the eight-cubic-foot icebox.

"We should be able to keep a dozen eggs," Merle said.

"More than you think. We can keep lettuce, fruit and the meat will last more than a few days!"

"Okay, you've convinced me. I'm sure glad we didn't come all the way over here for nothing."

"Let's head back," said George.

"Let me take a whiz first," said Merle.

"Good idea."

They loaded the icebox in the front of the boat. Merle pushed off and George pulled the starter rope. The dependable motor roared to life and George steered the boat out into the waves. They would have to head directly into the wind on the first leg. Then they would cut back around Red Cliff and after a short run, they would be on the lee side of Et-Then Island after they crossed Christie Bay. It was slow going into the wind, and Merle finally convinced George to back off on the throttle.

"Christ, my back is killing me!" Merle shouted.

"What'd you say?"

"Slow this son-of-a-bitch down!"

"We'll never get back if I slow it too much!"

"I don't give a shit!"

Merle looked at his watch as they turned with the wind along Ethen Island.

Seven o'clock and the sun was still almost straight above. George pointed to the clouds.

"That's the storm they were talking about. When we get around the island, we'll have an idea about the stretch run to the cabin. That wind will have almost 20 miles to roll and it will all be broadside."

Merle didn't need to ask what they would do if it was too rough. He'd waited out many storms while fishing in Canada. He knew you always had to respect the weather in the North country. As they reached the end of Et-Then, Merle knew they were in for a delay. The big rollers hit the rocks on the point and the spray spewed 20 feet into the air.

"We're going in right here!" shouted George.

Merle raised his eyebrows in acknowledgment.

They found a sheltered cove and beached the boat. Merle helped George out and together they pulled the boat up on the rocks. George took the rope and fastened it around the corner of the flat sedimentary rock. Merle picked up a couple of basketball-sized rocks and placed them on the rope. "Just to make sure," he cracked.

"Let's go up the hill and check the water on the other side," George said.

The ground was pitted with smooth stones as they walked past a tier of stunted spruce trees and up a short incline to the crest of the hill. The mosquitoes came at them from all sides.

Merle coughed as he inhaled a swarm of them and covered his mouth with his handkerchief. George took off his glasses and rubbed his eyes.

"Heaven save us!" started Merle.

"Mrs. Davis …" finished George. "When we get to the top, the wind will give us some relief."

It did. Together they looked across Hearne Channel to the far shore where the cabin was nestled. The sky was steel gray just below the sun and the sun was losing some of its luster. The lake was pitted with white-capped rollers.

"We'd need a cruiser to get across that," said Merle.

"That's big-ass water," said George. "We may as well settle in. We'll be here a while."

"With all those mosquitoes," Merle grimaced, "I don't have enough Crown Royal!"

"We'll build a fire," said George. "The mosquitoes don't like the smoke."

"Neither do I," quipped Merle.

"You'll like it better before long."

They went down to the boat, got their cushions out and looked in the shore box.

"Four apples, two candy bars, two Cokes."

"… and about four ounces of Crown Royal."

"I'll get some dried wood and start a fire," said George.

George was back in a few minutes. He poured a little gas on the wood and lit a match. Whoosh!! The fire was roaring immediately. Its warmth felt good. The mosquitoes kept their distance.

Merle lay down and shut his eyes. He hoped this wouldn't last long. He thought of his cot at the cabin. He dozed off.

It was the water running down his neck that awakened him. It was not really a rain, more like a heavy mist. It was getting colder. It was as dark as Merle had ever seen at Great Slave. He looked to the west. There was just a hint of light as the storm had blotted out the sun. George was asleep. He had propped his rain suit on three sticks to cover his head.

The fire was out. Merle was tempted to remove George's self-made shelter as punishment for letting the fire go out. He looked at his watch. Three o'clock. The wind hadn't slowed a bit. He went to the shore box and got his cup. He poured himself two fingers of Crown Royal. "Pretty good sipping whiskey," he thought.

He laid some dry wood on the fire. He blew on the coals. A flame broke out.

George sat up, "What's going on?"

"Just a pleasant night on the rocks with a hundred thousand mosquitoes!"

"Toss me an apple."

Merle grabbed an apple and eyed the last candy bar.

As George bit into the apple, the thought of the candy bar was too much for Merle. "George won't want it now," he thought.

George finished his apple and closed his eyes. The fire was smoldering and the mosquitoes continued to keep their distance. The mist had stopped. Merle closed his eyes and drifted off to sleep. His bird dog was on point. He slowly walked up behind her and reached down. "Steady girl." He kicked in the grass, his gun ready. "Are they running on you? Let's find them!!" The dog moved ahead 15 feet and then came down hard, her tail sticking straight up. Merle carefully advanced. "Steady girl." He saw a small clump of brush right under the dog's nose. He took his safety off and stepped on the edge of the brush …

"Wake up, Merle. Wake up," George shouted as he shook Merle violently.

"What the hell!" Merle grumbled.

"The wind has laid down. We've got to go. You were really zonked."

Merle stretched and staggered to his feet.

"Merle, this is a hell of a place to fish! It's about as good as I've ever seen, but I've been up here six times and I'm starting to feel the urge again. There's a nice lake a ways south of here. They call it Scott Lake. It's right on the southern border of the Northwest Territories. It's a little handier. I picked out a spot for my next cabin. We could partner up on the Scott Lake deal, if you like. First, I have to sell this cabin. All I want out of it is what I've got in it. Know anyone who'd be interested?"

"I don't know. Let me think about it. I might, yeah, I think so."

"What'd you say?"

"Bob Gollier is one of my best friends. He's a hell of a fisherman. He's a doctor in Ottawa. He has two sons and both of them love to fish. One of them even guided a couple of summers up at Great Bear. He's a doctor, too. He just moved back to Ottawa. He's a neighbor of mine. He lives next door to Tom Gleason, a lawyer friend you've met. Great big guy. Hell, they're all big guys. Bob, Bud and Tom have to weigh close to half-a-ton! Anyway, they all love to fish."

"Sounds like they like to eat, too!"

"I think I can put something together."

"Tell them I'll make the trip with them next year to show them the territory and how to stash all the supplies in the bush. "Oh, Merle, toss me my candy bar."

Merle swallowed hard. "I thought it was mine."

George's narrow face hardened.

"Oh, well, we'll be back at the cabin in an hour. Where do you want to fish today?"

"I think I'll take the day off. I deserve a rest on my vacation!"

When Merle got back to Ottawa, he presented George's offer to Tom Gleason and me. We agreed immediately to look at the cabin. We knew we could talk Rip Nesch and several others into forming a partnership if it looked like a good deal.

Tom and his son John and I went with George and his wife the next summer to look the cabin over. As we got off the plane in Yellowknife, our spirits took a sudden nose dive. An airline official came up to George and said, "Mr. Hary, I have bad news. We have a message that your son was killed yesterday in Los Angeles."

We told George how sorry we were and that we would help make arrangements for their trip home. George said quickly, "The wife will go bury him. I'm going fishing. The boy would understand."

When fishing with George or camping with him, you did it his way or not at all. He told you where to fish and how. He wanted each trout fillet cooked three minutes on each side, and a minute one way or the other wouldn't do.

George stashed all the supplies for his cabin in 55-gallon oil barrels that he had opened meticulously, cutting off the top with a hammer and chisel. He would then hide the barrels in the bush and cover them with pine boughs to conceal them. He left the boat next to the cabin, having an uncharacteristic trust of his fellow man.

We had a terrific week of fishing and decided that we would buy the cabin, as two other friends were interested in sharing the ownership. George showed us a list of his cost in the construction and supplies, including a boat and motor. His cost was $3,512.06. He told us he would like $3,562.06 and said the $50 was for his one-week labor and planning. As I wrote the check, I realized that the most important part to George was the six cents.

On our last day, George didn't fish, but stayed at the cabin. When we came back at noon, he was busily cutting out the top of another empty oil barrel with his hammer and chisel.

Sweat was rolling off his brow and mosquitoes were everywhere. All he said was, "I knew you boys would need another one of these!"

It amazed me that George and Merle could get along. They both were in the class of people who recognized there were two ways to do most things, their way and the wrong way. Merle would occasionally run into difficulty with a project and meet the adversity with a unique rationalization or a quick retort rich in the dry humor of a man who was determined to admit no failures. "Heaven save us, Mrs. Davis" and "Let the hide go with the hair" were two of his favorites. He would utter his one-liner with a palms-up gesture and a hint of a smile. He had the look of a man in a game of five-card stud with a trump as his hole card. Merle had just such a trump.

Some people are born with silver spoons in their mouths and providentially find help at the last minute to bail them out of disaster. Merle's trump card surfaced one summer when Merle had contracted with a pair of painters to paint his house. Merle had decided that a major project such as painting his beautiful two-story Dutch Colonial home in residential Ottawa should be let out to bids. He advertised in the classified section of the paper, and the low bidder started early one morning. By noon they had walked off the job, not appreciating Merle's constructive criticism of their performance, but savoring Merle's $50 up front earnest money.

"Neighbor, what can I do?" Merle asked Bob Soph across the alley. Bob remembers Merle was frantic. "I called Don Kornhaus, a friend and college classmate who had been in the Marines and was the high school track coach. Don and several teacher friends agreed to bail Merle out and finish the job." That was just the beginning for Don. The Sunday after they finished painting, Merle backed his car into his breakfast room. Luckily, Don was an accomplished carpenter and took care of Merle again after another frantic phone call. Don took such good care of Merle in Ottawa, it occurred to Merle he would be incalculable help on a fishing trip, so he devised a plan to move their act to the north. He was able to talk Don into going with him to his cabin on Scott Lake one summer. When Don came back, the stories flew around town hot and heavy.

The bears had been very active around Merle's new cabin at Scott Lake in northern Saskatchewan. The blueberries were scarce, so the bears were foraging more and were attracted to the cabin by the scent of bacon grease and food. On two occasions, the bears tried to force their way into the cabin at night. They seemed totally unafraid of humans, and because of their aggressive behavior, Don had to shoot two of them. Merle loved telling about the bear attacks and would roar when telling about doing dishes one evening when a bear stuck his head in the window.

"I just grabbed a skillet and pasted him on the snout," he would laugh. "Then he came around to the front door and met my man, Mr. Kornhaus, and his rifle."

The next year, Merle was looking for a new companion and enticed a card-playing friend, Jake Heck, to go along. Before he agreed to go, Jake checked with Don to find out what he might expect. Don prepared his instructions and handed them to Jake, along with a package addressed to Merle.

Jake read them to Merle at an impromptu gathering of friends at Merle's the night before they left. Tom Gleason, Bob Soph, Rip Nesch and I were all there with our wives. Don had asked Jake to present Merle a personal gift after he read the instructions:

INSTRUCTIONS TO ANY NEW FISHING COMPANION OF MERLE PRICE, HEREAFTER, REFERRED TO AS THE MASTER, ON FISHING EXPEDITIONS INTO NORTHERN CANADA:

(1) When traveling by car, don't suggest different routes to the Master even though it might be a shorter route.

(2) Be sure to get as many freebies on the plane as possible. (This really pleases the Master.)

(3) Do not criticize the Master for taking towels, soap and toilet paper from the motel on the first leg of the trip.

(4) Do not fail to boat any fish caught by the Master.

(5) Always have cold, fresh water ready for the Master's evening Nippy. (Do not criticize the Master for pouring a little extra Crown Royal into the glass. DO CRITICIZE him if he tries to have three "nippies", which he will.

(6) Do not complain when the Master maneuvers the boat so that he will have the first cast at an attractive rock or reef.

(7) Do not win too often at Gin Rummy when playing the Master.

(8) Devise ways to sneak Golden Nectar past the eyes of the border inspector.

(9) Always hold the boat steady until the Master is seated, or has disembarked.

(10) Be sure to loudly inform everyone you encounter that *your* guide is the Master.

(11) Perfect your ability to prepare fried mush.

(12) Do not make smart remarks about how many times the Master uses his bedside bucket at night. (It's better to say how hard it rained during the night.)

(13) Never catch the first fish of the day.

(14) Do not fry fish more than three minutes per side.

(15) When out on the lake, do not ask silly questions like, "Are you sure you know where you are?"

(16) Do not get your lure hung up more than the Master.

(17) Be sure to jump out of bed and start a fire before the Master arises.

(18) Do not panic when the Master is guiding the boat through shallow, rocky coves. (Best to close your eyes.)

(19) Do not expect the Master to help store equipment when preparing to leave for home.

(20) Tell the Master how good his stew turned out.

(21) Always stand between the Master and the bear.

Merle chuckled as Jake finished and held up the present he had unwrapped, a 5 x 7 picture of the Master at the helm of his boat at Scott Lake. The picture was framed by a hand-finished piece of hardwood. Merle grinned as he read the enclosed message.

THIS PIECE OF WOOD WORK IS CHISELED OUT OF FRANKLIN COUNTY, KANSAS NATIVE WALNUT. IT IS NOT PERFECT, NOT SQUARE, NOR WITHOUT MINOR FLAWS. THESE DEFECTS ARE INTENTIONAL. IT SHOULD HELP REMIND THE ONE WHOSE IMAGE IT HOLDS THAT HE IS NOT PERFECT EITHER AND THAT FOR ONE TIME HIS #1 BOY PUT THE BIG FRAME ON HIM!

ELEVEN

AFTER WE PURCHASED the cabin from George, I knew I had to take Dad and Mary Lynn to Robin Island. Mary Lynn was game for anything. She would go in a moment, but Dad was another story.

He had become much less sure of himself as his health failed, and to be abandoned in the wilderness for 10 days with no means of transportation to a hospital was stretching the lifeline just a shade too tight. As luck would have it, his cardiologist, Tem King, was an avid fisherman. Perhaps I could entice him to go with us, and if I could, I would have Dad trapped. I called Tem and made my proposal. He jumped at it and the trap was set! As I explained my plan to Dad, he recognized my intent, and the expression of a condemned man briefly crossed his face. Then he smiled and said, "Why not!"

To make the trip complete, we invited one of Dad's best friends, Bob Childs, an avid bass fisherman from Bryan, Texas. Bob was eager to share in the lake trout fishing up in the Arctic.

We had another problem that took some planning. We needed another boat at the cabin and would have to arrange to transport the boat 85 miles by air or 120 miles by water. A friend from home, Brad O'Dea, agreed to pull a boat up from Kansas City. It would be up to Brad and me to run the boat into our cabin with me as the navigator. That amounted to a 120-mile trip over uncharted water. I had fished 30 miles from the cabin, but the first 90 miles was to be a new experience. I trusted my summers at Great Bear would see me through.

It was going to be critical for me to view the first part of my route from the air on our flight into Yellowknife. The last leg of our flight was a short hop from Hay River to Yellowknife, and we hardly had time to stretch before we began the descent into Yellowknife. I had some very important work to do, and it was critical for me to sit in a window seat on the right side of the aircraft. I explained by predicament to a middle-aged, dark-complexioned man who worked for the Department of Fisheries at Yellowknife. I told him I was planning to take a boat from Yellowknife to a cabin on the east arm of Great Slave Lake and wanted to see the route from the air. He understood and we exchanged seats. I calculated that it would be 60 miles from Yellowknife to the Caribou Islands, which were less than five miles from the mainland. The critical turn needed to be made at Gros Cap between the point of the mainland and the Caribou Islands. I figured our boat, with a 600-pound load, would travel about 25 miles per hour. Barring an unfavorable wind, I planned to turn left two and a half hours into our journey. I wanted to make a visual inspection of the critical point where I would turn. I saw the Caribou Islands just past the point. Then I noted a deep bay, which could lead to a wrong turn just before the point. Another concern was unmarked reefs. I remembered the navigational rules in Ontario, never closer to the shore than 150 feet. Always pass black buoys on the left and red buoys on the right when traveling downstream. Of course, the converse is true when traveling upstream. Allow 75 feet on either side if a red buoy with a black ring. I had never seen a buoy on previous trips to Great Slave, but I had been well off normal navigation routes. I watched the water color carefully as we flew into Yellowknife and saw only one suspicious light yellow area. The reef was just between the mainland and an island with a prominent metal-roofed cabin on the north shore.

Otherwise, it looked as if my only concern was to stay a safe distance from shore. That had always been my habit in that country. I wanted to be as close to shore as possible in rough water. The Mounties, with the Air and Sea Rescue Squad, had told us at Great Bear that you can survive in that water for only three minutes. In rough water I made a habit of keeping as close as possible to shore since I can't swim very far in three minutes. The weather was calm. It looked as if the trip would be no problem. We arranged for Mary Lynn, Dad, Bob, Tem and Brad's wife Roxie to fly in by Twin Otter approximately two hours after we had left, and I asked the pilot to over-fly our route to ensure we wouldn't get lost. If my calculations were right, it looked like smooth sailing.

While shopping in the Hudson Bay Store prior to the trip to the cabin, Mary Lynn asked the checkout girl what the winters were really like. She stopped ringing up the sale and said, "Oh, about the first of October we all go to bed, and in the summer we divide up the babies." Mary Lynn laughed and smiled at me. Then she said, "I sound like a real tourist, don't I?"

The weather was a beautiful, bright clear day. As we put the motor on the boat and loaded up, the wind began to gust from the south. This could throw my timing off. The motor started on the first pull. Brad and I started out of Yellowknife Bay. I checked my watch and we were underway. The wind was not a factor, and 30 minutes out I saw the cabin with the metal roof and checked the area between the cabin and the mainland and saw an unmarked reef. Just as I suspected. I wouldn't have to worry about which side of the buoys to stay clear of.

At two hours, I began to look for the turn into the east arm. There was a point just ahead and I started a gradual turn, but before I completed the turn, I could see the high hills behind the bay, so we proceeded south. At two and a half hours I came to a point and made the turn. The sun was at our backs, and some 60 miles in the distance I could see the beautiful cliffs of Et-Then Island, which was directly across from our cabin. Suddenly I looked up and saw the Twin Otter carrying our wives and supplies. The pilot tipped the wings as they passed overhead. We arrived at the cabin at 11:45 p.m., and the sun was still high in the northern sky. As we made our final approach, Brad could not hide his sense of relief. He beamed at me and said, "You do a pretty darn good job of navigating."

"We were lucky the wind held off."

Mary Lynn, Roxie, Tem, Bob and Dad were all waiting for us as we beached the boat in the shallow bay in front of our cabin. After exchanging our hellos, I noticed the ground was littered with dried animal hides, hair and bones.

"The pilot told us all about it," started Tem. "The Indians used this cabin as their headquarters while following the caribou herd on its annual migration up through the Bathurst Inlet region on Canada's northern mainland coast to the summer calving grounds on the islands in the Arctic Ocean. They followed the herd with snowmobiles and ambushed them right here in front of the cabin. They dressed the animals here and radioed for a plane to come out on skis and land and haul the carcasses back to Yellowknife and haul whiskey back."

"We're lucky this is a dry climate." chimed in Mary Lynn. "There is no odor at all. There is an abandoned Indian village about 300 yards down the shore complete with tent stakes and drying racks and many animal skins lying around. That's where their families stayed. They cut the meat into strips and allowed it to dry on the racks. They then store it in bags for future use. The pilot explained how important the caribou is to the natives. Indians eat its flesh, make soup from its marrow and clothing and tents from its hide. They use the bones for needles, awls and knives and its horns for fishhooks, spears and spoons. They even use its tendons for thread. They don't waste anything."

We built a fire and burned the dried hides that evening, and the next morning the scattered bones were the only sign of the past winter's massacre.

A week in the wilderness in a two-bedroom cabin with five men was going to be an enlightening experience for Mary Lynn and Roxie. We allowed them the luxury of a private bedroom with the five men scattered from wall to wall throughout the rest of the cabin, Tem sleeping under the kitchen table. The women's private half-bath was a J.C. Penney catalog-ordered Porta-Potty, which was erected behind the cabin in the heart of the mosquito country, according to Mary Lynn. Bathing was innovative. Brad had the courage to wash in the lake and rinse off with 60-degree water. We took a Coleman stove to the flat rocks in front of the cabin and heated water to fill an aluminum bathtub, which was designed for a smaller species of man. My favorite method of bathing was the sun shower, which was a black plastic bag filled with five gallons of water that we hung on the south wall of the cabin exposed to the radiant heat of the sun. That warmed the water to a tolerable temperature and allowed me to rinse the Dead Woods Off and the musk oil that I had anointed myself with each morning to repel the monster mosquitoes that were everywhere. We were able to avoid the pesky insects inside the cabin and while on the lake fishing. The worst times were trips to the latrine, which could no longer be described as relief.

Brad was an ideal man to have along on such a trip. We had planned for Brad and Roxie to stay for three weeks and lend continuity for three different groups of four fishermen each. Roughing it in the wilds was not a new experience for Brad. He had been raised on a farm near Ottawa, one of seven children. Brad's home did not have indoor plumbing, but he was quick to say they never wanted for anything and always had enough to eat.

"We made do with what we had."

The difference between Brad and me was apparent one evening as we were fishing in the bay behind the cabin. We were casting where a small stream emptied into the bay. We saw a few oil drums and beached the boat.

"This is an old trail head," Brad said, "There must be a mine up along the stream."

Suddenly we noted two wooden pallets in the brush next to our boat. Brad exclaimed, "We can use these back at the cabin and make a fine dock for the boats."

It hit me like cold water in the face. I hadn't gotten past the realization that the pallets and drums meant that someone had been there previously, and Brad was already figuring out how to use what he had found. We took a rope and towed the pallets back and made a splendid, practical dock for the boats.

Mary Lynn loved the pristine country at Great Slave as much as I. It seemed there was always a loon, a bald eagle or a bear to observe.

One afternoon, as we were casting in a small bay across

from the cabin, a black bear ambled down to the shore. He had not seen us, and after a drink he turned and looked at us. He took a few steps and sat on a fallen tree and nonchalantly watched us fish. He didn't seem alarmed at all.

"He thinks he's a zoo bear," said Dad.

There was a small island behind the cabin with a huge eagle's nest in a large spruce tree in the center of the island. Using original thinking, we named the island Eagle Island and enjoyed watching the eagles feed their young as they stealthily watched us.

Mary Lynn loved the thrill of a battle with a fighting lake trout, and she performed as well as she had when crappie fishing in Arkansas.

I was running the motor one day with Mary Lynn in the front and Dad between us. Dad and I were casting and Mary Lynn was trolling. She hooked the first fish of the day, a beautiful 10-pounder. Dad released it for her, and soon she had another. Then I hooked a 12-pounder and Mary Lynn had another beauty. She was using a red and white Dare Devil and Dad had a silver one. I also had a red and white on, and as Mary Lynn hooked another one, I also had a strike. As Dad and I unhooked the fish, I could tell by the look in his eye he wasn't having any fun. He looked at Mary Lynn.

"How deep are you fishing?"

She smiled at him and said, "I've heard that before!"

"Let's trade lures," I said. "We don't have another red and white one in the boat."

"No, the lure doesn't make any difference. Sometimes it is the bow, sometimes it's the arrow, but usually it's the Indian!"

Dad kept watching Mary Lynn, and finally he looked at the water behind the motor. He pointed down and said, "Look at her lure, it's only about 4 feet behind the motor."

His voice trailed off as a large trout grabbed her lure and showed us his silvery side as he made his first run.

As I unhooked her 15-pound fighter, I unsnapped her red and white Dare Devil and replaced it with a silver one. Without a word, I placed the lure on the seat beside Dad. He had it on his line in a minute, and his mood blackened as Mary Lynn continued to pull them in and he continued to shoot blanks. He varied the speed of his retrieve, let the lure sink to the bottom and tried every trick he could think of. As noon approached, he said, "Let's go back to the cabin and grab a sandwich. Let me make one more cast."

Dad cast his spoon just off the shallow point where the waves were breaking and the turbulence and the spray had changed the clear water to a murky blue-green. As he began his retrieve, his rod suddenly doubled.

"Uh, oh, I'm hung up."

"Hold your line tight," I said, "it might be a fish. Don't give him any slack."

"No, it's solid. Try to run the boat into the wind a little ways. Maybe it'll pull off."

As I turned the boat, Dad's line suddenly got slack. He started reeling as fast as he could. When he picked up all the slack, the line was tight and running straight down under the boat. He set the hook instinctively, then held the line tight.

"Feels like bottom."

"No, it's moving. I'm holding the boat steady in this wind."

Suddenly the line sliced through the water toward the big lake. Dad smiled and raised his rod tip. The stiff six-foot fiberglass rod was bent in the manner that not only said "Fish," but "Big Fish." Dad loosened the star drag, and I pointed the bow of the boat into the wind and followed Dad's fish.

"He's going down," I said. "He's a big one. We'll let him play himself out in the depths."

"I'm glad he didn't stay in the shallows with all this wind," Dad said.

Suddenly Mary Lynn yelled, "I've got another one!"

Her lure had been trolling behind the boat, and she had forgotten about it with the excitement of Dad's fish.

"You're on your own, Babe. I've got my hands full with the boat in this wind, and Dad's got all he wants."

Mary Lynn kept reeling, and her reel hummed as the fish stripped line on his first run.

Dad's line still pointed straight down.

"I gained a little line a minute ago, but he's just twisting and turning in a circle down there."

Mary Lynn sat down and looked at me disgustedly. "Bud, you've got to do something." Her line suddenly got slack.

"He's off, thank goodness."

She quickly reeled in and set her rod beside her seat.

"I'm quitting. I'll just watch you two."

Dad was watching his line intently.

"I'd just like to see this devil."

"Watch out!" Mary Lynn shouted as she noted we were drifting close to the rocky shore as the wind picked up. I headed the boat back into the waves, and as I turned we caught a big swell on the side and a wall of spray soaked Dad and me in the back of the boat.

"Thanks, I needed that," Dad said as he wiped the water out of his eyes with his right sleeve. His left hand had turned white as he held onto the rod and tried to hold the rod tip up to keep pressure on the fish. He braced the rod with his right forearm to rest before trying to regain some line and entice the fish to move off the bottom.

"At least we don't have to worry about getting the line caught in trees as we do when fishing in Arkansas. I'll just have to let him wear himself out. I hope he wears out before I do."

Time had gotten away from us. With the sun never setting, it was no help in estimating time, but my stomach said it was late.

"I think he's coming," Dad said. He lifted up on the rod with his right hand, then quickly reeled in the captured line, careful to always keep the line tight.

"Don't horse him," I warned, repeating the advice he had given to me thousands of times in southern Canada.

Dad's face continued to show the strain and concentration.

"Whew, my back's about to give out."

"Hang in there. You don't have much line out. We ought to see him pretty soon."

The star drag screeched as the fish made another run. Dad stopped him and turned him.

"I hope that was his last one. He's not very deep."

"There he is," I yelled as the big trout rolled on the surface. "He's got moss on his back an inch thick."

"He's coming toward the boat, Bud. Watch the motor!"

"I've got to keep us off the bank."

"I know, but watch my line. That monster is coming under the boat. I know you don't have a net. Do you have a gaff?"

Dad knew I didn't like nets because half the time the hook would catch in the net and jerk the hook out of the fish's mouth. Once netted, the fish would twist and turn and the net would be impossibly fouled and would have to be cut free.

"No," I said simply.

"I was hoping. How the hell do you get the big ones in the boat?"

"I don't know," I smiled. "I've never boated one."

"You'd better get this one in the boat."

"You just bring him along side carefully and I'll figure something out."

"You'd better. He'll go 30 pounds."

"Fifty, if he gets away."

Dad stood up in the boat and winced as he hyper-extended his back.

Mary Lynn took a towel out of the shore lunch box and wiped the perspiration from his face.

"Thanks, dear."

We were drifting closer to shore and the wind had died down slightly. I looked at the back of the bay we had dubbed Oso Negro Bay for the black bear Dad had sighted. There was a small rocky beach protected from the big rollers by the point where Dad had hooked his fish.

"Keep him in close. We're going to beach that whale!"

The fish obediently came into tow alongside the boat about two feet down. It was then that my heart skipped a beat.

"He's just barely hooked in the side of his mouth. With all that twisting he has almost torn the hook out. We had better move to that beach."

As we neared the beach, the fish started moving away from the boat. I decided it was not time to dally.

"Keep him in tow," I said to Dad, "We're going in!"

I didn't vary the speed, but just headed straight toward the beach scarcely 40 feet away. As we got into the shallows I tilted the motor up. Dad sat down preparing for the jolt when the boat hit the beach. He handed me the rod. I turned away.

"You keep the rod, he's your fish. We'll just lead him up onto the beach."

I turned to watch the fish as the lure came loose. I didn't have time to think. Luckily, the fish was exhausted. The water was only four feet deep, and I had the beautiful fish cradled in my arms before I thought what I had done.

"PoPo isn't here to pull me out this time."

The fish took our 28-pound scales to the limit, and we estimated his weight at 33 pounds.

"Let's shoot a few snapshots and turn him loose," Dad said. "I think he's done."

After the pictures, I put him in the water and quickly thrashed him back and forth through the water to move some water through his gills. He slowly began to stiffen, then his pectoral fin moved and his tail began to wave. He began to move. I grabbed at his tail, and he started slowly swimming toward the depths. We watched him until we could see him no longer, careful to look for that tell-tale flash of white that signaled he was going to belly-up, but he stayed down.

Dad enjoyed taking charge of the cooking, as he had no peer as a gourmet cook in the North country. At the end of the week, as we circled the cabin in the Twin Otter for one last look prior to our flight to civilization, Dad looked at me and said, "I've never seen anything like it!"

TWELVE

To ESCAPE THE STRESS of a busy physician's life, Mary Lynn and I would often take off and travel the country roads to enjoy the peace and quiet of Mid-America. We would often stop by a farm pond for a few minutes of fishing and relish the time to ourselves, away from the telephone, with the only sound the rustle of the wind drifting through the trees and tall prairie grass or even an occasional bird's whistle or distant cow's plaintive bawl to punctuate the quiet. One day Mary Lynn said, "You know, we should buy a small farm, something we could call our own."

I called a realtor. Before I knew it, he was at the front door. We spent most of the day looking at rural property. I was looking for a 40 or an 80-acre piece of ground with a small pond loaded with bass and crappie. Most of the places he showed us were improved with a home and outbuildings or were too large for our budget. Finally he showed us a place that was really rough. It was about five miles from town and was bordered on the south by a small creek. It was an irregular piece overgrown with thorny hedge trees. On one corner was an 80-acre field of pitifully thin milo interspersed with weeds.

"If there's ever a market for hedge balls, that place will be a gold mine." I told the realtor.

"The owner would let it go on contract, and I think she will sell it right."

"How big is it?"

"Four hundred and sixteen acres. She wants three hundred dollars an acre."

"I'd have to have three partners to afford that, and I don't know if there are three other crazy people around."

Mary Lynn and I walked the entire farm early one morning. We were walking into a slight easterly wind along a ridge

116

banked by a grove of walnut trees. The sun was just beginning to caress the native grass on the ridge as it crept over the tall cottonwoods in the ravine that led to the creek. Suddenly I heard a crash and saw two does dart out of the thicket and run down along a small stream to escape into the timber along Middle Creek. As long as I could remember, the sight of wild game had been enough to restore my faith in freedom and unbridled free expression. A deer, a flock of geese, ducks, a fox or any creature in the wild is free to do just what they want without the constraints of civilization. I knew after seeing those two does that I would have to find a way to buy that farm! I showed it to several friends, but they just scoffed.

Then I showed it to Bo Killough, the son of a very close friend. Bo was 12 years my junior. He worked for his father in a construction business, but had helped his grandfather on his farm since he had been a child. I had admired Bo's boundless energy, as he always had some project going. In addition to working for his father and helping his grandfather at the farm, he always made time to plan a party for a charity at which he served as the disc jockey. In his spare time he was either jogging or planning some new endeavor. All these activities perplexed his father, who felt there was enough work to do in the construction business to keep him busy, but Bo was a dreamer. When he looked at a project, he could see past the obvious. He could see the full potential and look past, or over, as his father would say, the obstacles.

I showed Bo the farm one day, and we walked from one side to the other. After we were done, Bo said, "Come with me."

We climbed into his truck and went to his grandfather's and drove through the pasture.

"See this red clover? It puts nitrogen back into the soil. We can get lime from Killough, Inc. after we get the soil samples tested. We then have to build terraces and waterways and it has to be fenced. I can get a dozer from the company and we can clean out a lot of that hedge. That will improve the pasture."

"Bo, we ought to talk to two other people. I figure we could spread the risk and it's big enough for several people to enjoy. We could dam up the ravine and probably have a 20- to 30-acre lake!"

"Whenever you build a dam, you must consider what you're covering up. We could lose a lot of grass and trees."

"I know two other guys who might be interested."

"We don't need cautious partners. Let's share this dream together."

We bought the farm and called the partnership the K-G Development Company. We enjoyed hunting quail and squirrel, and one Thanksgiving day Bo, John and I, along with my brother Fred and nephew Bill, were hunting when we were shocked to see a flock of 50 wild turkeys slowly browsing through an early winter wheat field.

During the winter when Middle Creek froze, our entire family enjoyed ice skating and sliding around on the ice. We would park the car along the road next to the low-water bridge that crossed Middle Creek and then walk along the creek the entire length of the south border of our property. Game tracks were everywhere.

After spring planting, we would make weekly trips to the farm during the growing season to see how the crop was doing, or rather not doing.

We met Bo one evening at dusk. The soybeans were just beginning to bloom. We parked behind Bo's truck and met him at the fence.

"It's a pretty good stand," I said.

"Yeah, but the price is awful," said Bo. "We'll have a good crop, but we won't make any money."

"We never do."

Mary Lynn saw the gathering storm on the horizon, "We'd better get back to town."

We could hear the thunder roll in the distance.

"Things are going well." I said to Mary Lynn as we got back into the car.

"We have a lot to be thankful for. The kids are growing up."

"Sharing this farm with Bo is a special experience," she said. "He is always on the go."

Mary Lynn looked at the dark thunderheads as the wind began to kick the dust of the gravel road. The storm was coming fast with a lot of noise and lightning.

"Yes, things are indeed going well," she said. "It's been a beautiful evening. That storm looks mean. I hope it's not an omen."

"We need the rain."

"You always try to find something positive in threatening situations."

"There are two sides to every coin."

"Unless it stands on edge."

"Mary Lynn, it makes a lot more sense to be mindful of the positive things, while preparing for the worst."

"Murphy's Law again, huh?"

"I guess so. We're going to beat the storm home."

"I hope so," Mary Lynn said as she cast a worried look at the clouds.

BOOK TWO

Above the Pons

THIRTEEN

IT SEEMED an insignificant injury. I fell backwards while adjusting my ski boot and landed on my right elbow. I had a sudden pain in the right lower back that subsided in a few seconds. Although my back was tight, the crisp morning air and newly fallen snow were too tempting and I spent the day trying to keep up with my family on the Breckenridge slopes and even skied Mach 1, an expert slope, in a very cautious fashion. That evening my back tightened, but I felt a heating pad and two aspirin would suffice.

The next day we made the trip home and I was able to resume my usual routine. I would jog one and a half miles each morning and then make hospital rounds prior to a full day in the office. I gradually began to note some nausea associated with a headache. I had my blood pressure taken at the hospital one morning and some blood tests run by our laboratory. My blood pressure was 140/96, which was just at the upper limits of normal. However, I had jogged to the hospital that morning and felt that may have accounted for the mild increase. All the laboratory tests and a routine urine analysis were normal. Because of the persistent nausea, I had a gallbladder X-ray, which was also normal. The discomfort persisted, but I wasn't going to let it get me down.

I played volleyball one evening and noted the onset of a slight headache. It had been three weeks since my skiing injury and my back was no better. Things at the office weren't going well either. Dave and I had worked hard to recruit a new young physician to join us and reduce our work load and share night call. A physician fresh out of the military had agreed to terms and had moved to town the year before and had built a big practice, but he was having marital problems and his wife had asked for a divorce. He was leaving town. That meant a marked increase in my work load. We immediately scrambled to find a replacement, but prospects were slim.

One morning I went out to the farm with an agriculture extension agent to survey plans to put in terraces and waterways for erosion control. We had to walk over some uneven terrain and climb up a small rocky bluff. I slipped once and again felt a sharp pain in my back. We returned to my car and got stuck on the way home. Pushing the car out of the mud didn't help my backache, and when I got home, I decided I had had it! I grabbed my fishing rod and told Mary Lynn I was going fishing that afternoon. My father and I went crappie fishing at a nearby pond. The headache seemed to get much worse, and after an hour of fishing, I asked Dad to take me home. When we arrived, I decided I had been doctoring myself long enough and Dad took my blood pressure, which was 230/130. We called Dr. Chuck Ford, who had been my personal physician at Metropolitan Hospital, and he arranged an Intravenous Pyelogram (I.V.P.), a kidney X-ray, for the next morning to see if a kidney problem was causing the high blood pressure. A shot of Demerol brought some relief, and the next morning Dad picked me up for the trip to the doctor.

The Intravenous Pyelogram was done by Dr. Hamilton, who had previously been the consulting radiologist at our county hospital and was well known to my father and me. As he put the one-minute film on the view box he stated, "Looks pretty good." But I noted a delay of visualization on the right side, and my father agreed. The delay suggested something was obstructing the flow of dye through the artery.

Dr. Hamilton said, "Maybe there is a little delay on the right." The next clear memory I had was of Dr. Bill Lee, a neurologist and medical school friend in my hospital room and Mary Lynn with a worried look on her face.

A spinal tap had just been performed by Dr. Ford, and I was nervous about the results. I wondered if I had had a stroke.

I looked at Bill and said, "Did I bleed?"

He looked down at his shoes, then at Mary Lynn and said, "I guess that says it all."

I fell back on the bed, and all consciousness left me. It

was chilly. There was a breeze coming through the screen windows above the lockers. I had goose bumps. I was shivering. I needed to dry off and warm up, but all the towels were wet. They were scattered about the concrete floor. Not a dry towel anywhere. I went to look for the attendant. There was no one there. I went to the door. It was locked. I picked up the phone. It was dead. I walked back out to the pool. The door was locked.

I looked through the glass. There was no one in the pool. The lifeguard was gone. It was getting colder! I tried doing jumping-jacks to warm up. Where was everyone? That was the substance of my subconscious. I could not escape that bath house. I screamed, and no one came. I couldn't understand what I was doing there. I don't like to swim.

The next four weeks were mostly blank. I remember Mary Lynn and brief interludes with concerned friends and the bath house. The vague realization that I had been in the medical intensive care hovering near death came slowly.

One day Dr. Ford explained carefully that I had had a blockage of the right renal artery as a result of a tear after an injury. My blood pressure had been uncontrollable, and after a hypertensive cerebrovascular accident, due to a hemorrhage of a ruptured artery, I had part of my right kidney removed. They had saved the lower half because, luckily for me, I had an extra renal artery on the right side.

"It was really a screwy case!" he said.

FOURTEEN

DURING MOST of my hospitalization, the question was one of survival. The physicians caring for me in intensive care during the early phase told my family my chances of survival were bleak. They were giving little hope that I would wake up. This has caused me to explore the reasons for my survival. Psychologists have studied the "survivor personality" and have determined that people who survive best gain strength through adversity. They turn inward for personal strength. People who lack the survivor qualities tend to look elsewhere for help. The survivor personality has been described by Salvatore Maddi, Ph.D, of the University of Chicago, as having three components: (1) A sense of commitment to and involvement in your life, (2) A feeling of control over your circumstances (and the willingness to recognize what you can't control), and (3) The ability to see change as more a challenge than a threat.

Jacob Lindy, M.D., of the Cincinnati Psychoanalytic Institute in Cincinnati, has stated that survivors are better able than others to make sense out of what happens to them. "They have the flexibility and ego strength to integrate even a terrible experience into the rest of their lives so it seems to have meaning." These people simply believe in the value of their own lives and life itself.

According to Bruce Bohrenwend, Ph.D., professor of social sciences in the department of psychiatry at Columbia University, the support of other people vastly increases the odds for survival. He suggests maintaining strong attachments to people and causes. "Those who have strong commitments, clear values and things to believe in are less likely to become disoriented and break down in a crisis."

There is no question the support of Mary Lynn, family and my community was instrumental in my survival. The dedication to the principles instilled in me by my parents and my church have provided a clear direction for the rest of my life. I had been relentless in my pursuit to see that there would be some benefit as a result of my misfortune.

Once I survived the physical threat, there was a psychological trauma to overcome. My very existence was challenged and my life had taken a new direction. My confidence was going to be tested. Could I depend on inner strength to overcome my disability, or would my disability pose a threat to my ability to function effectively? Nancy Moss, Ph.D, in a paper titled "Conservative Responses to Severe Psychological Trauma," stated that people who adjust to severe psychological trauma have strong personalities and are goal oriented. She has written that a creative response is often common to these people. They share determination that some good will come from their misfortune, and they tend to develop new talents to make up for their losses.

There can be no question that I have been blessed with many of the characteristics of the "survivor personality." My family and my experience during my formative years provided me with the mettle and sense of purpose to overcome long odds. It certainly helped to have the Lord on my side when the going got tough. However, I was also the recipient of some old-fashioned good luck. The major damage inflicted by my stroke was to the brain stem. Vision and hearing were the only senses that were affected. The higher central nervous system functions were preserved. Because of the peculiarity of human neuro-anatomy, I was left with attractive choices.

The pons varolii produces a prominent swelling with well-defined borders on the ventral surface of the brain stem between the medulla oblongata and the cerebral peduncles of the mid-brain. Above the pons lies the cerebellum, the thalmus and the hypothalmus. The thalmus serves as a relay station for the sensory stimuli to the cerebral cortex and has important integrative functions.

The higher levels of the human experience — reason, commitment, faith and decision making — are centered above the pons. The development of these mental processes effectively separates mankind from lower animal forms. The development of the intellectual faculties has led to the capacity for man to decide to survive and, in fact, to will survival, physically and psychologically. When lower pathways are affected, function is impaired, but with preservation of the higher centers, new skills can be developed selectively to compensate for the losses.

FIFTEEN

I HAVE BEEN ASKED many times to describe the feelings of frustration and humiliation associated with the rehabilitation. Didn't I feel degraded by the therapy? Not at all. I was an object. Therapy was security. I was not aware of my condition, and I needed the comfort of people to take care of me and tell me what to do. It would be natural for an observer to think I would feel humiliation and frustration as he can relate to the normal human condition. But I was an object in a total stimulus-response state. I had no initiative at all. I was not humiliated or frustrated because I was not able to comprehend the difference between me and others. I could not relate to normal functional capacities. I was taught in six months to function in a manner that had first been programmed nearly 38 years before. I had to learn to feed myself, dress myself, climb stairs, write and address personal hygiene needs. When I had my first session with the occupational therapist, she asked me to write my name. I took the pencil and began in my barely legible scrawl — which was improved — B-U-D-D-D-D-D — then the therapist had to take the pencil from my hand, "That's very good, Bud!"

Mary Lynn says I was very task-oriented and would follow instructions very well for the only time in my life. Never was my lack of initiative more apparent than when returning from therapy one morning with Mary Lynn and Dr. Sampson, the chief of rehabilitation medicine at Metro. The elevator door opened at my floor and Mary Lynn and Dr. Sampson stepped out, but I stood in place with the others as the door began to shut.

Dr. Sampson turned and said, "Bud, your patients won't understand when you don't get off the elevator at the proper floor."

Once I started something, it was hard to get me to stop. I

was very repetitive and was eager to please people by doing the job exactly as instructed. I could perform tasks successfully, and this enabled me to build and improve my performance. Every new successfully performed task was a monumental occurrence. I was very compliant, and Mary Lynn insists it was a blessing as it would have been very difficult for me to progress had I been hostile and physically aggressive and resisted any effort to direct me.

Therapy was very tiring. The past was a void, and only the sight and sound of Mary Lynn would bring that past into focus and help me set goals for the future. I had been reduced to the functional state of an infant and had to climb all the way back. I had to be totally reoriented to the roles of adult, husband, father and, finally, physician. Mary Lynn remembers:

> *A major victory was Bud's transfer from medical intensive care to a regular hospital room. The cubicle in the I.C.U. was so sterile. There was nothing visible unrelated to life support. We were so alone, yet we had no privacy, but we did not need privacy. A nurse or doctor was always there and looking through the open doorway with a direct line of vision to the central nursing station. I was reassured to know they were so close. The beep, beep, beep of the heart monitor was endless! The rhythmic cardiac monitor was interrupted only when Bud would turn or raise his hand and play with the wires.*

> *Sometimes I thought he did that for orneriness. But he wasn't in a mood to be ornery. We were very careful about visitors. I felt he should have company even if he didn't communicate with them. Dr. Ford disagreed. If people see him like this, rumors will be all over Ottawa. I felt it would be worse if we didn't allow any visitors at all. There were some I couldn't refuse. Bob Soph and Merle Price fished with Bud many times and they promised not to stay long. Tom Gleason was able to get the best response from Bud. He came into the room wearing a bright blue fishing cap with a polar bear*

logo. Bud had one just like it. It was his favorite cap. He and Tom had gotten them at Great Slave when they had fished together. Bud smiled, rubbed his eyes and said to Tom, "We'll have to do that again sometime."

Tom and I smiled at each other with tears in our eyes.

Gradually, Bud entered more into conversation, but he didn't initiate much. When his office nurse came to call, he addressed her by using the name of a nuisance patient they heard from daily.

When we got to the regular hospital room, the visitors were harder to control. One of Bud's patients from Ottawa was in the hospital on the same floor. He was in our room twice a day. The visitors consistently encouraged Bud and expressed faith in his recovery. Buzz and Sue Kelsey, both high school classmates of Bud's, were there all the time. Not just to see Bud, but to check on me and see if I needed anything.

Larry Forsythe visited several times. He would talk Bud's legs off about the "good old days." Several of his fraternity brothers called to encourage him. The support was overwhelming!

The rehabilitation was tedious — speech therapy, occupational therapy and physical therapy. I had a therapist for everything. One was even assigned to my bowels. After a few weeks, I became competent in self-care and was dismissed to continue my convalescence at home. As a final test in rehabilitation, Dr. Ford asked me to explain diabetes to him.

"Diabetes mellitus is a metabolic disease characterized by deficiency of insulin, which is required to transport glucose across the cell wall where it can be utilized to provide energy. If there is not enough insulin available, the glucose accumulates in the blood stream and the body uses alternative sources of fuel, such as fat and protein, to provide energy. First the liver supplies glycogen, which can be converted to glucose, and finally fat may be broken down and used by the cell. This results in weight loss and accumulation of ketones in the blood stream, which can produce acidosis. This may lead to diabetic coma. The first step in management is diet control and weight loss, and if this is unsuccessful, insulin administration may be required. It is critical that the diabetes be controlled as diabetics are at high risk of heart attacks and stroke ..."

"That's enough, Bud," Dr. Ford interrupted. "I don't think there is anything wrong with your ability to think."

My primary handicap was in visual perception, thanks to a large defect in my peripheral vision as a result of the stroke. I also had a central hearing defect and a problem with translating visual and auditory input into appropriate verbal and motor responses, which resulted in a sluggishness and a problem at times in recognizing acquaintances and putting a name to them immediately. This was a talent I had always enjoyed, and the delay was to become a source of frustration for me. The solution to this disability was simple enough, but not easy to accept — be patient, take time to be sure and respond appropriately and at times explain the disability to others.

One day Mary Lynn and I were sitting at the breakfast table drinking coffee when Mother drove into the driveway. She walked in and had a cup of coffee. I was glancing at the sports page of the paper. Mother suddenly said, "It's 10 o'clock in the morning. Most men are at work. Bud Gollier, the Lord did not spare you to sit around and drink coffee."

The message was clear. It was plain her remark was born out of love for me. It was time to move on. I had a debt to pay to those who had pulled for me.

After talking with several physician friends and having them quiz me, I was satisfied that my intellectual and judgmental functions were intact. And now the big question began to loom on the horizon — could I go back to my practice and would my patients accept me?

After a few weeks at home, it became apparent that financial consideration aside, I had no talent as a homebody. I can remember many times my father saying he had a deal with the bankers ... he didn't lend money and the bankers didn't practice medicine. I had the same deal with the plumber, electrician, painter, auto mechanic and carpenter.

In short, I was a complete dud as a helper around the house. So now the question was when to return to work? My partners had been perfect during my convalescence, but were eager for me to return. Delores Edwards, my loyal office nurse, was especially encouraging. I got the okay from Dr. Ford and started back half-days six months after my stroke. It went well and my patients were very understanding. Nearly all of my previous patients returned to my care, save only a few who had developed a relationship with one of my partners. This did not concern me, as this happens all the time in partnerships when someone is covering during vacation or days off.

Three months later I was working full-time and taking night calls. The only problem I had was with depth perception as a result of the visual field defect and, as a result, I was insecure with complicated lacerations and episiotomy repairs in obstetrics.

My partners agreed to back me if I was uncomfortable with the laceration repair, and I reluctantly decided to give up obstetrics. All went well other than frustrations with my vision's effect on my golf game.

I also decided to give up quail hunting after an experience at a controlled game reserve. Tom Gleason and I had our bird dog on point and, as I stepped into flush the quail, I heard the familiar flutter and saw nothing! Then Tom said, "He's on to you," as the bird escaped into my visual field defect. I then realized that a hunting companion could be walking in my blind spot and I didn't have any business carrying a gun ...

He makes it sound so simple! So now the question was when to return to work. I didn't want to inappropriately push him, but he seemed very comfortable just doing nothing. When he got home from the hospital, we planned a walking program, but it was like pulling teeth to accomplish it and to establish a discipline. He seemed to enjoy the boys' ball games and would go with the children and me to play a few holes of golf. The boys were amazed how well he played and hit the ball most of the time, but it wasn't straight down the middle and he had trouble following it and would throw the club down and say, "I just can't play this damn game. I can't do anything!"

Initially he would lie in bed looking at the ceiling and wave his left hand next to his face to see if his vision was returning. At first he couldn't believe what had happened to him and would insist his vision would come back totally. He just wouldn't believe he had had a stroke.

I finally talked him into doing some swimming at a neighbor's pool. That lasted six days. One morning he broke his fifth toe on a lane-dividing rope while swimming. When he came home he said, "You might as well get me a room in a nursing home!"

His recovery progressed from plateau to plateau. He would seem comfortable for a while and then a new challenge would cause him to withdraw. He would maximize potential difficulties in any new setting. He displayed a firm belief in Murphy's Law, "If anything can go wrong, it will." It was frustrating to see him fail to initiate the necessary climb to full recovery. I tried to get him to read medical journals, but he couldn't get involved in those either. They continue to pile up in his office. I encouraged male friends to come over to stimulate him to a more active life, but they seemed uncomfortable around him.

Perhaps he reminded them of their own vulnerability. "There, but for the grace of God go I."

I finally decided I was going to have to push a little harder. I reminded him that the disability checks weren't going to put his children through college, and he slowly began to talk about his practice.

Driving was also a problem. His central vision was 20/20, but he had to be very careful at intersections. The occupational therapists had all stressed that he needed to work on being more aware of his left side. I would ride with him, and he was always careful to look to the left two or three times at all intersections.

Five months after leaving the hospital, Dr. Ford and he agreed he was going to try it at work. We decided at *first I would drive him to make hospital rounds and then to the office. Picking him up at the office was really depressing. He would get in the car and seemed very discouraged. But in talking with his partner and the girls in the office, I could tell they felt he was doing better. He was his own worst critic! He missed obstetrics, but I could tell he was enthused about his hospital practice.*

One morning three months later, as I waited outside his office, I was dreading to hear his usual self-deprecating remarks. He came out and opened my door on the driver's side and said, "Scoot over, chauffeur, you're fired. We've got to play the cards we are dealt. I may as well quit complaining and make the best of it!" From that point on, he was much happier and he felt more independent. He was more interested in family activities and mentioned his disability only rarely. He began to talk about skiing again and started making plans to take the boys to his cabin in the Northwest Territories. That had always been one of his dreams. Making plans for the future was a sign that he finally believed he had to be concerned with more fulfilling things than his immediate needs.

SIXTEEN

BROTHER FRED was the key to my dream of taking my boys to the cabin in the North. Fred shares my passion for the outdoors, and we had been planning a trip before my hospitalization. I felt I could pull my share of the workload on such a trip, but Fred would be a great help when the boys were ready to go. Fred had never been to Great Slave, so we put together a trip two years after my stroke. Fred and I flew to Yellowknife, the capital of the Northwest Territories, the day before the rest of our party to check the cabin and boats since none of us had been there for four years. It was fortunate we decided to check as one our boats was missing. The cabin was in great shape, and we had some good luck when we reported our loss to the Mounties. One of the Mounties said he had seen a green boat on a beach 15 miles from our cabin the day before. We flew out to the beach and sure enough, it was our boat. It had been "borrowed" by one of the natives.

The fishing trip was a great success. It is hard to beat the thrill of catching 8- to 20-pound lake trout casting in shallow water.

One evening while sitting around the cabin after I had fixed chowder, Fred was describing my illness to our fishing companions. He said when he visited me in the I.C.U., I would just mumble "East Mizzonquin, East Mizzonquin, East Mizzoquin." He asked what East Mizzonquin was. Everybody was amazed that a person who had been that sick only two years before would function so normally. They were amazed I could remember where all the reefs were. The depth perception problem slowed my pace when going down the rocky, boulder-strewn path from the cabin to the boats, and I was careful to wear leather gloves when cooking or unhooking fish. I could tie a fisherman's knot in the dark by feel, as I had done that since I was eight years old. I was a little slow, but I didn't get hooked or burned. My perceptual problem surfaced only once. Although I had no fear of getting lost, putting distances and times together was difficult. Our companions were always asking how far a fishing spot was from our cabin, and I said everything was 20 minutes away. It made no difference whether it was 5 miles or 30 miles. That became quite a joke until we nearly ran out of gas one day on a 20-minute trip for a little Arctic Grayling fishing at a spot that was actually 30 miles from the cabin.

The next day we really got into the lake trout. They were feeding on ciscoe, a bait fish, in shallow water on a windy shore behind the cabin. The three of us in my boat had about two hours of fantastic fishing. We all had fish on our lines at the same time several times. There was no telling how many fish we caught and released. I was just sick that Fred and his two companions were missing the action. We decided to go find them when we all had our lures in the boat and had caught our breath. We found them around the first bend and told them where to go as they had had a slow afternoon. We went back to the cabin to rest and start dinner. The wind began to blow harder. Three hours later, I started to worry. The wind was still blowing, and I have always felt both boats should fish together in case of motor problems or worse. We loaded up and went to the hot spot to look for them. They weren't there, and I really started to worry. I remembered losing Huck and Hi at Great Bear, and I remembered George had always cautioned us to respect the water. "That's big-ass water out there!" George would say.

Suddenly I saw a speck way down the shoreline. We hurried down there, and I was relieved to see three of the biggest smiles I've ever seen! Fred said they were just worn out, and they had caught fish on nearly every cast since they arrived. I smiled back and said, "You like it here at East Mizzonquin?"

The next year Fred and I had the thrill of our lives sharing the experiences with our sons, Bo and Bill. On Bo's first day on the lake he caught several trout on our way to a shallow bay where northern pike spawned early in the summer.

George had dubbed the bay "the snake hole" because pike are a narrow fish with a long, toothy snout. The action is always fast if the pike are spawning in "the snake hole." Bo was excited as we headed into the bay. He had heard Mary Lynn and Big Daddy talk about their experiences there.

On his first cast, a six-pound pike hit his line and jumped completely out of the water. Bo's mouth dropped open.

"Wow!!"

His line went limp as the fish spit the lure out.

"Darn!"

He threw his spoon right to the edge of the weeds and began his retrieve. Suddenly his rod lurched and he nearly lost it. He eyes widened and his reel screeched.

"I've got one, Dad!"

I grabbed the movie camera and started taking pictures. Rip Nesch, who shares my love of the North, was in the front of the boat.

"You'd better put that camera down. Bo's gonna need some help. He's got a horse!"

Bo wasn't saying a word. He was holding on for all he was worth and was intently looking in the direction of his line. Suddenly, the big pike rolled on the surface! He had a big white belly and looked to be as long as the canoe paddle in the boat. Rip and I were both giving Bo lots of advice, but he acted like he was ignoring us. I lifted Bo's first pike into the boat. We weighed him quickly, took a few pictures and Bo released him. The fish sped away, but his memory will never leave. Seventeen pounds of fighting fish. Bo threw another cast and hooked another monster, almost exactly the same size. I unhooked him at boat side, after confirming his weight — nearly 17 pounds. Bo threw another cast and hooked another.

"Dad, I've really got a horse this time," he said excitedly.

"What the hell," I thought. "He's just caught back-to-back 17-pounders and now he thinks he's got a horse!"

The fish did seem to be pulling harder. Rip and I looked at each other quizzically.

After another long fight, we lifted an eight-pounder into the boat. He had been hooked in the tail, giving him more leverage, and that explained Bo's anticipation of a bigger fish.

One evening Rip guided Bo and me into another East Mizzonquin experience. After an hour of catching fish one after the other, Rip finally tired of taking Bo's fish off the hook and releasing them. He told Bo he was on his own as he hadn't boated a fish of his own since we started, and we were giving him a hard time about "wearing the collar." Bo handled it perfectly, and Bo and I had fish on at the same time frequently. Finally Rip said, "Enough of this father-and-son treatment. Let's go back to the cabin, I need a beer."

Bo and his cousin, Bill, ran the motors, prepared shore lunch and helped with all the hard work associated with a wilderness adventure. Bill's quest for the huge trout he had seen and hooked briefly one day became an obsession. I've never seen anyone fish so hard and long. He even named the fish SEF for Someone Else's Fish.

As I was filleting the last of the morning's catch to give to the pilot and crew as a token of thanks for their friendly service, Bo took the fillets to wash them in the cold, clear water. He looked at me and said, "Dad, you didn't tell me it was going to be this good."

Fred and I agreed after the trip that we had taken two boys to the North and returned with two young men.

Two years later, it was John's turn when he reached age 12. He could hardly wait to go northern fishing as he had heard all about his brother's successes. When we entered the "snake hole" where Bo had caught his big fish, John was having problems with his reel. He had one backlash after another and caught only one small northern. His face was getting longer, and after one of many backlashes, I could detect tears welling in his eyes. The disappointment in John's heart was apparent by his facial expression. The poet must have had John in mind when he coined the phrase, "wearing one's heart on his sleeve." It is as if John has a talking face. When he is satisfied with himself in any endeavor, he wears a smug, confident, happy look, but when he is unhappy, his face clouds over like a sudden thunderstorm.

It suddenly occurred to me that we were a week earlier than usual, and since the "snake hole" was much warmer than the rest of the lake, there might be some lake trout seeking the warmer water at the mouth of the shallow bay. It was easier for John to cast the heavier Rocket Devil we used for lake trout, so we moved to the opening of the bay. John made the first cast, and his rod bent double as a monster trout hit his lure. His reel hummed as the fish stripped his 20-pound test line. I started the motor and John held on for dear life. He kept as much pressure on the fish as he could and slowly began to make progress.

When the big trout was first sighted, John smiled, "Wow, did you see that?"

After what seemed like hours, I was able to lift John's fish, an 18-pound lake trout, into the boat. John's face told the whole story. What a cure for the backlash blues! His brother was going to hear all about this one! We took some quick pictures, and then John carefully lowered the fish into the water and grabbed his tail and gently gave him a shove. The beautiful fish swam slowly a few feet, then suddenly, realizing he was no longer restrained, swiftly fanned his tail, sending spray across John's face. Then he was gone to thrill someone else another day.

The fishing at Great Slave Lake is only part of the thrill. The country is like a frontier. Although it is beautiful, it is far from tranquil. It gives me a sense of movement, of action. I can almost feel the glacier move. Across from our cabin are 300-foot cliffs that make up part of the longest continuous fault in North America. There are many beaches along the shore in that area with large, smooth rocks the size of basketballs strewn all along them. Then periodically there will be a finger-like glacial till composed of sedimentary rock with large, smooth rocks mixed in as the glacier had tilled the bottom out of the lake. The flora is typically alpine and the native wild flowers are beautiful. The rocks along the shoreline are covered with bright orange, yellow and red lichen, which give the impression that someone had passed through with a paintbrush. With all the water around, it is hard for me to believe that the annual rainfall is similar to the Sahara Desert. The pine trees tell the story of the barren dark winters. The pines exposed on the north shore and north sides of the islands are stunted and shriveled with sparse needles. However, those on the south shores with the greater sun exposure, are taller, sturdier and much greener.

As I stood on the front of our cabin looking at the cliffs of Et-Then Island 13 miles away, I would almost hear George say, "Be sure both boats always fish in the same area. That's big-ass water out there!!"

With Rip, John and me was Scott Carder, a psychiatrist from Los Angeles, who had been in medical school with me and Bob Soph, and his son, Chris, who were neighbors from home. Although Chris was eight years older than John, they had crossed paths a time or two, and Chris had even babysat for us when John was a baby. Bob was a confirmed fisherman, and Chris would rather fish than anything he could think of. We fished three to a boat with Rip and me serving as guides. That gave everyone a variety, because Rip and I had two different philosophies on fishing and we both thought we were right. Rip was committed to fishing windy points and preferred trolling and then casting and drifting with the wind when he found the fish. There is nothing wrong with that method if you like bass fishing or beer drinking, but if you are after lake trout, you need to remember they are going to be seeking the ciscoe, their primary prey in the food chain. Fish are cold-blooded and therefore seek temperatures rather than conditions or bottom structure. The ciscoe and lake trout are more active in the 53-degree to 58-degree range; therefore, there is going to be more action in the warmer water right after the ice goes out. The warmer water is going to be in the shallow bays down the lake from our cabin.

We have learned this over and over on our fishing trips. These lakers have not actively fed all winter, and as soon as the ice breaks and the water warms, all hell is going to break loose, but not on those windy points.

One day coming back from the "snake hole," we stopped in a shallow bay and Bob made a cast into the murky shallows just off a beach. Suddenly his reel screamed and he almost lost his rod. The trout made a run at the beach, and Bob hadn't even engaged the reel as the fish was just stripping his line. I could see the line cutting through the water toward the woods behind the beach.

"Where's he taking you?" I said to Bob.

"Wherever he wants to go," he said quietly.

Bob said several times during the next few minutes that he had never had a fish pull like that one! Finally we lifted him into the boat, and then Chris had one off the front of the boat.

"This is almost as much fun as catching carp on corn at the Second Street dam," Chris joked.

Both fish were in the 20-pound class, and I had two confirmed shallow water fishermen in my boat.

Scott had gone to high school in North Kansas City and had patterned his early adolescence after James Dean's character in "Rebel Without a Cause," a popular movie in the mid-1950s that had served as a premonition of the protest movement of the 1960s. He had been a member of a street gang and had won his first car in a poker game. In college, Scott had become relatively civilized as he had concentrated on his number one priority — his studies. His passion in social settings was analyzing other people's behavior. Therefore, it was natural that he would be attracted to psychiatry. He was very comfortable offering an opinion on abnormal behavior because he was satisfied that any deviation from his behavior was abnormal. Occasionally, his past would surface.

One morning I went down to the boats to gas up before going fishing and Scott followed.

We brought our gas in by plane in 55-gallon drums. On past trips we had wrestled with the drums so that we could pour the gas into the cans with the help of funnels. It was hard work for two men, and we had planned to buy a pump for this trip. I priced them in Yellowknife, and the best price I could find was $150. I then bought an eight-foot hose and decided to siphon the gas, thinking I could suck a lot of gas for $150. As I sucked on the hose that morning and the gas came close to my mouth, Scott suddenly grabbed the hose and said, "Let me show you how to do that." He grabbed the hose and threaded it into the barrel. Quickly he put his thumb over the end of the hose and lowered it rapidly to the opening of the gas can and took his thumb off. A steady stream of gas poured out. Scott's quick glance over his shoulder did not escape me.

"Who are you looking for, the cops? You've siphoned gas before, haven't you?"

"I've got an aquarium at home," he said quickly and flashed a smile. A subsequent visit to Scott's home in Los Angeles resulted in a diligent search that failed to locate an aquarium.

Later in the week, we went past the "snake hole" to an abandoned gold mine for a tour. Touring the mine was Rip's specialty, and he took the boys and Scott on a tour while Bob and I went around the corner into a very shallow bay where I hoped the northern pike would be spawning just as they were in the "snake hole." Sure enough, they were there. We caught four or five in a row, and then I suddenly remembered one of my father's favorite lures for northern fishing. The problem with catching northerns is unhooking them as they flop all over the boat. It is hard to unhook them without hurting them or getting a hook in the finger or worse. Dad thought he could have just as much fun if he took all the hooks off a Lucky Thirteen, a floating wooden bass plug that had always been on of his favorites. We had always pinched the barbs down on our hooks, but it was still dangerous to have a frisky northern in the boat with a treble hook in his mouth. Dad would throw his lure out on the water and pop it a few times. Soon there was the thrill of the strike and the brief battle before the fish let go. Then an amazing thing happened! An eight-pound northern grabbed the lure and wouldn't let go. Soon he rolled over and the wire leader slipped behind his gill plate. A few minutes later Dad had him in the boat. It had been said that a sportsman fishes with barbless hooks, but a true sportsman fishes with hookless lures. As I clipped it onto my nine-inch wire leader, Bob looked up and said, "You're not going to try that, are you? I've heard all about that, and that has to be the world's biggest fish story!"

He watched intently as I spun the hookless lure over the top of the water. I popped it a few times and the water beneath it exploded. After a brief tug, the lure floated to the top. I made eight or 10 more casts without a hit, and then I had several fish in a row grab the lure, but quickly spit it out. Bob started razzing me.

"How long are we going to play this charade?" he said.

I then looked at him and feigned disgust.

"I forgot the trick. Dad always lassoed them."

In a moment I had another hit. I pretended to throw a loop across the water with my slack line and said, "Come along, little doggie!"

As luck would have it, the fish rolled over at that time and the leader slipped behind his gill plate and the razzing suddenly stopped. As I led the 10-pound northern along the side of the boat, Bob said, "You're really going to put that son-of-a-bitch in the boat, aren't you?"

"You bet your sweet ass," I said as I lifted the fish.

We went to meet Rip, Scott and the boys after their mine tour, and Chris and John begged Rip to take them northern fishing. Rip winced, but agreed. Scott went trout fishing with Bob and me, and we told Rip where we would be, knowing an hour of catching northern was all Rip could stand, as he was a dyed-in-the-wool trout fisherman.

We went back toward the cabin a few miles and fished for trout. We weren't having any success, and after three hours we got worried and went back to look for the other boat. As we passed the mine, we could see Rip's boat slowly pulling out of the northern bay. The boys were all smiles, but Rip looked pretty grim.

"How many did you catch?" I asked.

Rip held up this bloody hands and pretended to count the wounds.

"Ninety-six," he said quickly.

Then I could tell he had cleaned each cut with a little beer and poured the rest down his gullet. The fishing continued to be excellent the rest of the week.

Scott couldn't believe there weren't any people around. "It's not like Los Angeles. Wait till I get the word back to the City of Angels. This place will be packed next year."

The last day of fishing was another beautiful day. As we went down to the boats, I told John I would like to fish with him the last day.

"Who's going with us, Dad?"

Bob had been in my boat the day before, and he suggested that Chris go with John and me the last day. Chris was in my boat in a flash, and as we pulled away, Bob smiled and said, "I feel like I just got shipped down to the minors."

We had another fantastic day and joked all day about being on the A-Team. Rip, Bob and Scott had the biggest fish of the day, so no one was disappointed. The conversation at dinner that last evening was full of fish stories and reminiscing about a fabulous week of fishing.

Scott was animated. He had caught the biggest fish of the day, a 15-pounder. As he was recounting his fish stories, as fishermen do, I interrupted him.

"Scott, when I was guiding at Great Bear, I discovered the guests fell into two categories. One group was composed of veteran fishermen who understood the slow times and were very patient and enjoyed themselves immensely. It took me most of the summer to understand the other category. They were complete novices. Many had never been fishing before. They would have brand new rods and reels, new outfits and new L.L. Bean boots. They were after a trophy or a picture to show a neighbor or relative who had bored them too long with fish stories. It has been great having you on this trip, Scott. Who are you trying to shut up?"

"My brother-in-law. He's always talking about the great trout fishing in Montana. Now I can do a little talking too. I've been trout fishing."

The next day we packed and were waiting by the shore at noon, which was the scheduled arrival time for the airplane. The boats were out of the water by the cabin and we all had a very satisfied feeling. As the Twin-Otter came in from Yellowknife and touched down on the water in front of the cabin, John looked at me with a tear rolling down his cheek and said, "I don't want to go."

Scott was taking pictures of our departure and put his camera down long enough to say, "I wish I could capture this and bottle it. I could be the busiest psychiatrist in L.A."

SEVENTEEN

I KNEW the question was coming. After the Christmas holiday season, spring break is next on the calendar, and spring break is the time to go skiing in the Colorado Rockies. The first year after my illness, Mary Lynn and I arranged for Bo, John and Sara Jane to go to Winter Park with the church group. We all had great memories of our family ski trips. It came out of the blue after I carved the turkey on Christmas Day. As I was serving the turkey, Sara Jane said, "Dad, are we going skiing this year?"

"We'll have to see," I said.

"You know, Bud, we ought to go at spring break," Mary Lynn said.

"I don't know if I could ski."

"If you don't go this year, you never will."

"I'm afraid my problem with depth perception will make it dangerous to ski the moguls."

"You don't have to ski the hard stuff. Just cruise down the mountain on the green slopes."

"It might be a real disaster."

"Remember when we skied with the minister at Vail on the 'Meet the Mountain Tour?' He had us blindfold ourselves and ski down the mountain by feel so we could sense how a blind skier feels. You didn't have any trouble then."

"I guess you're right. Let's do it!"

"The kids will be thrilled!"

The skiing went well. On the last day, Mary Lynn and I were enjoying a run down a gentle slope at midday. We came to a junction and stopped to enjoy the beautiful winter view of the Rocky Mountains. Mary Lynn pointed down to the right. It was a wide intermediate, more difficult slope. The trail had been scarcely skied that day, and the eight inches of morning powder was mostly undisturbed.

"Look, no one is skiing on that slope! It's so peaceful. Isn't it beautiful?"

"I thought the one we were skiing was beautiful."

"Oh, come on." And off she went.

"Oh, what the hell," I muttered as I followed her down the mountain. We went from side to side at an even pace. I followed her lead, turning on the moguls just as she did. We were able to control our descent safely. We got to the bottom without a stop, and neither of us was out of breath as we prepared to ski down to the lift line.

"You did that really well! You didn't even stop once."

"I had to keep up with you. Did you notice how crowded that slope got as soon as I got on it?"

Suddenly we heard a yell from Sara Jane, Bo and John, who burst out of the trees to our right and above us. They skied straight at us at an alarming speed, judging the distance between us carefully so they could be certain to spray us with snow as they skidded to a parallel stop. Sara Jane's smile lit up her sunburned face.

"We've been skiing behind you. When you left the easy slope, we went to the trees. It was a ball!"

EIGHTEEN

MERLE PRICE returned from an early September fishing vacation at Scott Lake one year and told me he had had some weakness in his left arm and leg one evening after a long fishing day. He thought perhaps it was due to a strain associated with running the motor. He said for a few hours he had no grip at all in his left hand. I examined him and found him to have normal strength in his left arm and leg. His neurologic examination was within normal limits, but when I listened to his neck with my stethoscope, I heard a loud bruit or murmur over his carotid artery.

"Merle, you need to have that looked into," I said, trying to hide my concern.

"It'll be okay. I just got a little tired fishing and overdid it a little."

"Don't give me that. You need to see your city doctor right away. It might be serious. I'll call him for you."

"I'll call him," Merle said. "I'll do it this week."

"You better!"

Merle went to the city and was admitted to the hospital for tests. When he got home he called and said, "They said I have a little blockage, but there's nothing to do at age 82. They told me to just take it easy."

Dad and I discussed it and agreed they didn't understand Merle very well. They needed to know he planned to hunt quail every day during hunting season and spend at least two weeks every summer in northern Canada. Merle did not think of himself as 82. Dad called Merle and told him we wanted to encourage his doctor to look at him again.

That night Merle had another spell with weakness in the left arm and leg. He rushed to the city. The next morning I went to see Merle at the hospital. I saw his doctor in the hall outside his room. As I explained Merle's activity level and was trying to point out a stroke is devastating at any age, the doctor interrupted and said, "Merle had a stroke last night. It happened at home after dinner." We agreed Merle might have had the stroke with the surgery and his age was against him.

As we were walking out of the hospital, I said to Mary Lynn, "Merle and I have something in common other than love of the North."

....

Over the six years following my illness, a few disconcerting thoughts had bothered me. Mary Lynn and Fred implied that some funny things had happened at Metropolitan Hospital. Mary Lynn said she had been at my side the day of the stroke and I was mostly ignored by the floor nurses, and when I had the seizure, the nurses didn't know who I was.

"Who is this patient? Who is his doctor?" they had asked.

She said they were like the Keystone Kops. Fred said Dr. Ford seemed very upset about some nurse who will be "taken care of!"

One day Mary Lynn asked whether I wanted to look into it. I dismissed the question curtly by saying, "No, they don't make mistakes at Metro!"

But the nagging doubts persisted, and I began to question the hospital.

One day it occurred to me that I had been admitted on Friday morning and the stroke was on Saturday evening. All I had was straight-forward renovascular hypertension, a Goldblatt kidney, that I had learned about when working on dogs in physiology lab as a freshman in medical school. We put a clamp on an artery to the kidney and the dog's blood pressure shot up dramatically. The increase was due to the fact that the kidney sensed the change in pressure due to the interruption of blood supply and released a hormone, renin, which acts to produce a potent vasoconstrictor, angiotensin II, which raises the blood pressure.

I had been assuming the stroke had occurred shortly after admission. What had happened in those 36 hours?

On the sixth anniversary of my stroke, I called Dr. Ford and told him that I had some hard questions to ask relative to my care. Had some nurse ignored an order? Dr. Ford was taken aback, but then recovered and assured me that I had first-class care throughout my hospitalization. He knew nothing about any problems with nurses. He told me my blood pressure was normal one hour prior to my stroke and that I was on Nitroprusside by intravenous drip. He also said he would be glad to go over the entire chart with me at any time. After repeating the conversation with Mary Lynn, she insisted that not only had I *not* had an intravenous, but I hadn't had any special attention from the nursing staff, even after the spinal tap, which was done three hours prior to my stroke. I then asked for copies of the hospital chart to include the admitting history and physical, progress notes, consultations, laboratory and X-ray reports, as well as Dr. Hamilton's I.V.P. report.

"A pre-admission hypertensive I.V.P. was normal," read Dr. Ford's admitting note.

Dr. Lee's consultation stated, an "I.V.P. on the day of admission was reported as normal."

The kidney specialist who took charge of my case in the Medical I.C.U. after the stroke dictated, "An I.V.P. before admission was reported as normal." Didn't anyone look at it? Where is Dr. Hamilton's report? Then I found it.

"There is prompt bilateral and equal visualization of the Nephrograms. The kidneys are normal in size, position and configuration, etc. ..." I had read this type of report hundreds of times! This is called a standard normal dictation in the trade. The kicker was that it hadn't been signed by Dr. Hamilton, but by his partner. Dr. Hamilton apparently hadn't had time to dictate a report after viewing the film with me and my father.

But had Dr. Ford not looked at the I.V.P.? I look at every X-ray and laboratory test I order. Had they suspected the I.V.P. may have been abnormal on Friday, the day of admission, I might have had prompt surgical intervention and been spared the stroke!

After the chilling revelation, the chart became more interesting. The CAT scan of my brain was normal. I had a barium enema on Saturday morning. Bowel tumors can cause blood pressure problems. Following that, I had a spinal tap, which revealed an opening pressure of 300 millimeters of water, nearly twice normal. The closing pressure was 106, and Mary Lynn says Dr. Ford told her, "We have to get his blood pressure down."

Dr. Ford realized this increased cerebrospinal fluid pressure, associated with hypertension, could be life-threatening. Fred was in my room at that time and he insisted Dr. Ford said something to the nurse about "a double IV or an IV in each arm." Still I was in a regular hospital room with no special attention, not medical I.C.U.

Mary Lynn had related that I had rested fitfully for several hours after the spinal tap and seemed very uncomfortable.

> *.... No one seemed very worried, but I could tell he was miserable! Everybody seemed to think his headache was the result of stress, but it wasn't any better after 24 hours of bed rest. I wanted to ask the nurses to call Dr. Ford, but I didn't want to be a nag. This was Bud's hospital. They knew what they were doing. Besides, what did I know!! Finally, I asked him if the headache was getting worse. He stood up and screamed, "I can't stand it!!" Then he fell on the bed and started shaking all over. I thought he was dead! Am I a widow?*
>
> *I screamed as loud as I could and two or three nurses came in. They looked puzzled and looked at each other like they were the Keystone Kops. One said, "Who is this patient?" The other said, "Who is his doctor?" They both left and then a resident came in and checked Bud and said he would call the attending doctors.*

It was then Dr. Lee came in and concluded that I had, in fact, had a brain hemorrhage. After a short time, Dr. Ford rushed in. Mary Lynn said he seemed very upset and personally escorted me to the medical I.C.U.

My care in the I.C.U. was excellent. Many of the nurses were friends and acquaintances from my residency, and they were a source of great comfort to Mary Lynn during my long stay there.

The review of my record was a chilling experience, but

what am I to do? What's done is done. I am now recovered with minor, but permanent difficulties. I am practicing full-time in a slightly modified fashion and enjoying my service to my patients.

Perhaps some of my colleagues would insist that, because I am a physician, I should not question my care at Metro. I had not asked for the doctor's orders and nurses' notes. I would need to review the entire chart and Dr. Ford's records.

In the medical profession, one must never stop learning from experience and improving. In every case, judgment predicates a particular course of therapy. This judgment is based on observation, examination and evaluation of the responses to the course of the therapy. We must depend on the nursing staff to help us evaluate the response to therapy. I have had a number of experiences wherein I wish I had chosen a different approach. When the results of my care are unexpected or unfortunate, I examined the course and ask what I might have done differently in order to have changed the outcome. Unfortunately, we cannot turn the clock back. Hindsight is always 20/20, but we must never stop trying to improve.

How could Dr. Ford say my treatment had been first class all the way when I had gone into the hospital with an acute hypertensive crisis and had a stroke 36 hours later? It was apparent that he and I had totally different perspectives about my treatment. There was nothing to gain by talking with him until I had reviewed all the records to my satisfaction.

I visited with an attorney, a friend of mine, who suggested I request the records from Dr. Ford, Dr. Hamilton and Metropolitan Hospital, but that the statute of limitation had probably run out as far as recovery through litigation was concerned.

The records from Dr. Ford came promptly and confirmed that the I.V.P. was reported as normal. Then a consultation from the kidney specialist revealed that I had not been on the Nitroprusside by intravenous drip until after the stroke. Mary Lynn defended Dr. Ford's faulty recollection by saying, "It's easy to forget things you don't want to remember."

The hospital chart would tell the story.

NINETEEN

"It is much easier to write upon a disease than upon a remedy. The former is in the hands of nature and a faithful observer with an eye of tolerable judgment cannot fail to delineate a likeness. The latter will ever be subject to the whim, the inaccuracies and the blunders of mankind."

— *William Withering*
(1741-1777)

TWO DAYS LATER, I received a call from the attorney's office. My chart had arrived in the morning mail. My heart was racing as I drove to town to pick it up. Would I find out that my care had, in fact, been first class? Dr. Ford had been right about the X-ray. What about the nursing care and the doctor's orders? I quickly scanned the doctor's progress notes. Nothing out of line there. Then came the doctor's orders. I had not been given any potent blood pressure medication, but Mary Lynn had said Dr. Ford felt my problem was due to stress, and with the normal X-ray, his decision to sedate me with Librium could not be criticized very strongly. I was interested to see how I had responded. On the first day, my blood pressure had remained high in the range of 190/110 according to the flow sheet, which recorded the blood pressure every eight hours. On the second day, the day of my stroke, my blood pressure at 6 a.m. was 190/120. The nurse's notes would reveal what my course had been on that fateful day. The note at 6 a.m. indicated I had complained of a headache, but had had a quiet night and my blood pressure was 200/120. And then a blank.

"Son-of-a-bitch!" I muttered.

"What's wrong?" I hadn't seen Mary Lynn slip into the den.

"There aren't any nurses' notes from 6 a.m. until I was admitted to I.C.U. at 6 p.m.

"I've been trying to tell you there wasn't any nurse."

"Oh, Mary Lynn, you just don't understand hospitals. Sometimes we are so busy we don't have time to chart. You know there were nurses' notes somewhere. It was an emergency."

"They didn't even know who you were!"

The next note was at 6:15 p.m. and stated — "Admitted to Medical I.C.U." During the most critical 12 hours of my life I had had no care at all. Fred and Mary Lynn had been right. During those 12 hours I had a barium enema, a CT scan of my head, a spinal tap, a consultation with Dr. Lee and a stroke, but I had not had a nurse. An aide had recorded my blood pressure at 190/110 on the flow sheet at 2 p.m., and my blood pressure was 240/140 at 4:50 p.m. and at that time I was given a blood pressure lowering agent in the vein. That must have been after I had the seizure as a result of the ruptured blood vessel and stroke. Thereafter, my blood pressure was taken every five minutes until I was taken to the I.C.U. by Dr. Ford. I would have been just as well off at home. Mary Lynn was the only nurse I had.

It was apparent that the convulsion and Mary Lynn's screams had gotten the nurse's attention, but what had my blood pressure been after 2 o'clock? Dr. Ford had ordered a strong diuretic, a water pill, to reduce plasma volume and increase urine output after he left my room, and the medication sheet indicated it had been given at 2:10 p.m. But my blood pressure was not taken again and there was an "X" marked through the output blank on the fluid balance sheet. The nurses had not notified Dr. Ford that there had been no response to the water pill, and there was no evidence they had an idea what my blood pressure was doing. The nurses obviously weren't aware I was in the hospital. If the nurses had been aware my blood pressure was going up, they could have notified the doctors and I might have been treated aggressively because it was apparent that a conservative approach wasn't working. There was no evidence Dr. Ford had checked back to see if the blood pressure that "we just have to get down" had responded to the diuretic. Then at 4:10 p.m., just 40 minutes prior to my seizure, I was seen in consultation by Dr. Lee, who described my headache as "essentially unchanged" since admission and that I was "incapacitated" by it. His dictated consultation stated I had had intermittent central flashing red lights of non-formed objects and then a normal CT scan of my head and the elevated spinal fluid pressure. Under the examination he stated, "He appeared uncomfortable from his headache and vomited twice during the examination." He then described a totally normal neurologic examination, but he did not record my blood pressure. He concluded I had a headache secondary to hypertension and suggested "medical management for now," but he was describing hypertensive encephalopathy.

According to the Sixteenth Edition of Cecil's Textbook of Medicine, "Hypertensive encephalopathy is an uncommon neurologic disorder characterized by headache, nausea, vomiting, visual impairment and focal or generalized seizures, which may proceed to stupor or coma ... Hypertensive Encephalopathy is a medical emergency. Its treatment consists of the prompt lowering of the blood pressure, taking care to avoid dropping it to hypotensive levels. The drug of choice is Sodium Nitroprusside administered parenterally. Although the intracranial pressure is commonly raised, it will respond to lowering of the systemic pressure and separate therapeutic measures are not required."

Twenty minutes after the seizure, Dr. Lee was back in my room, and his progress note indicated that my examination at that time suggested a brain stem cerebrovascular accident. As I studied this report, my mind suddenly jolted back to my third year in medical school. The chief of neurology was discussing spinal taps, and he was going through the entire procedure step by step. He emphasized the importance of measuring opening and closing pressures and reporting the volume of fluid removed. Then he said, "After the needle is in place, remove the stylette carefully. If the fluid spurts out indicating increased pressure, put the stylette back in quickly and be very careful about how much fluid you remove or you may herniate that patient's brain stem through the foramen magnum at the base of the skull, and then you will really be in a pickle."

Next I looked at the CT scan done the day after my stroke, and everything suddenly came into focus. "Since the study yesterday, there is now increased density around the brain stem — particularly on the right side high up. This is associated with some enlargement of the lateral ventricles."

At that time, I checked Dr. Ford's note on the spinal tap to determine how much fluid had been removed. There was no mention of the volume of fluid removed in his note. I checked the pathology report to see how much fluid was received by the laboratory. Once again, there was no mention of the volume of the fluid analyzed.

In order to have such an unfortunate result, there had to be a failure at all three levels of responsibility in the health care delivery system. The primary care physician had to lack communications with the nursing staff and his consultant. The consultant had to fail to follow through with his recommendations and to communicate with the primary care physician, and the nursing staff had to fail to record the vital signs and lack of response to the diuretic and to communicate this information to the physician.

It was apparent that none of the three were meaningfully involved, but each of them must have assumed someone else was in charge.

TWENTY

THE REVIEW OF MY CARE in the Intensive Care Unit reflected the first-class care Dr. Ford had talked about. For six days, my blood pressure had been taken every five minutes, then at least hourly for 20 more days. The nurses' notes revealed much of the horror Mary Lynn had endured. My hallucinations and deliriums were vividly documented. Often I was discussing medical cases I had had in the past. On one occasion, the nurses described me talking "with someone named Rip" and wanting a radio to go to my cabin to listen to the weather report. Once again, I was escaping the reality of my perilous state by dreaming of a fishing trip. Rip and I would often listen to the weather report on the radio to avoid being caught in a storm. On other occasions, I would be calling to Mary Lynn or the children. Numerous doctors were involved in my care as my blood pressure was a constant problem. Initially, intravenous medication controlled it, but then that became less effective. Then a dye study of my kidney circulation was performed and revealed the blocked artery. Surgery was then scheduled and the top half of my right kidney was removed. However, my blood pressure did not dramatically return to normal and then the intravenous medication became ineffective. There was increased pressure on my brain and Dr. Lee inserted a pressure gauge through my skull to monitor the pressure, and powerful drugs were given to reduce that pressure. Finally, it was determined that the increased pressure on my brain was causing the resistant hypertension and I was given a general anesthetic to bring the pressure down. This was effective, but what an effort by the medical team!

Slowly I began to respond to conventional medication, and my level of consciousness improved. During this period, there was some concern that I was blind. Friends asked Mary Lynn if I knew who she was. She said she thought so, but hadn't had the nerve to ask.

Finally she got up her courage during a period when I was more responsive. She asked if I knew who she was.

"Sure," I said quickly, "Claudine Longet!"

In her words...

> ... *The long hours of waiting in Bud's room, hoping for some encouraging response from him, gave me plenty of time to wonder about our future. How will the bills get paid? The children needed Bud so much. Will I have to start looking for a teaching job? Fred was a great help at this time. He took charge of our financial affairs. He called Bud's office manager and found out about his disability insurance policies. He was reassuring and relieved my mind so that I could devote all my energy to helping Bud get well.*
>
> *One of the visitors from home, Dr. Bill Ballinger, a psychologist at Ottawa University, had emphasized that it was critical for me to talk to Bud in a very positive way, just as I always have. He would say, if I couldn't be positive, I should stay away from him.*

Although my remark must have been a cruel blow to Mary Lynn, there is no question in my mind that I knew very well she was a person very important to me. She was always offering encouragement, telling me about home, the boys' baseball games or Sara Jane's dance lessons. She was forever keeping me in touch with reality. She went to every rehabilitation session with me and never wavered from the positive attitude that I would make it back all the way. This was a long ordeal for her, but her grief was eased by a magnificent community while I was in the hospital. The prayer support was overwhelming. There was a community-wide healing service and prayer vigil one noon at our church when I was in the middle of my darkest hours. It was then that the doctors thought I was blind, and at noon, as the prayer vigil began, my mother was in my room in the I.C.U. She got up to get a drink of water, and I suddenly looked up and said, "Hello, Big Nelle."

From that time on, my hallucinations and deliriums were less frequent. Every minister in town called on me at least once, and they all helped keep my family in great spirits. Although my medical care at the time was excellent, Mary Lynn's unremarkable positive attitude and continued support from a community that never stopped offering its prayers had an immeasurable impact on my recovery. The community support kept Mary Lynn going during our darkest moments. My recovery was considered by many to have been a miracle. It is apparent that I had the help of the Great Physician.

... He had absolutely no idea how sick he was! He was in a coma for most of a month! He rambled on unintelligibly most of the time. Occasionally, he would mutter my name or call to one of the children. He also talked about his cabin on the Great Slave Lake on several occasions.

He would call the name of his office nurse and mention a medical term and seemed to be dictating a medical chart. His weight loss was shocking to me!

I could not believe my healthy and robust husband, so full of life, was wasting away in front of me. His arms were black and blue from the endless blood pressure checks. He was constantly pulling at the intravenous tubes and the catheter and wrist restraints that were required. The 48 hours on the breathing machine, under anesthesia, were almost too much for me. I made small talk with the anesthesiologist while wondering if my husband was going to wake up.

The children initially stayed with their grandparents, and I would give them nightly reports, but they were too young to understand. Sara Jane was only six, John was seven and Bo was nine. They knew their father was very sick and I tried to be positive with them. I would tell them he asked about them and wanted me to kiss them good night for him. I would tell them he was getting better, but I wasn't sure. He had a lot of attention in the I.C.U. and there was little I could do. He was in their hands.

It was after the prayer vigil at our church that he seemed to get better. He seemed to be more aware of people in the room and began to take food by mouth, but I had to feed him. The intravenous tube was finally removed. It was when he called me Claudine Longet that I began to see light at the end of the tunnel. On our ski trip, which now seemed like years ago, we had seen the message on the blackboard at the chair lift. "OLYMPIC SKIER SPIDER SABICH SHOT IN ASPEN BY CLAUDINE LONGET." To call me Claudine was the devil in him and I felt a weight coming off my shoulders. He still had his sense of humor.

After a few weeks, the children had to be home in their own beds. They missed their pets and needed to get back into familiar surroundings. I had a sitter spend the day with them while I was at the hospital. Finally, we made the move from I.C.U. and back to a regular hospital room.

There was progressive improvement, but everyone was shocked at the 60-pound weight loss.

Finally, Dr. Ford and I agreed that NO VISITOR signs should be placed on the door. We were afraid everyone would comment on the weight loss and intermittent confusion and rumors would abound at home.

The children were anxious to visit their father. One weekend I took them to the hospital. I decided he should be dressed in street clothes rather than a hospital gown. None of his pants would fit, but a couple of safety pins fixed that. I got him dressed and took him to the lobby in a wheelchair. When he saw the children, he smiled and slowly stood up, and he stretched out his 6-foot, 6-inch frame — minus the 60 pounds — John jumped up with glee and said "Wow, Dad's a real basketball player!"

TWENTY-ONE

Matthew 7:12

RELIGIOUS TRAINING came in pieces and was mostly developed from isolated experiences.

Among my earliest memories are those of Mother coming into my bedroom to kiss me good night and "tuck me in." She would then lead the prayer that she taught me to pray:

Now I lay me down to sleep. I pray the Lord my soul to keep. If I should die before I wake, I pray the Lord my soul to take.

I can remember being frightened at times by the thought that God, the benevolent Father, would take my soul to Heaven any night he wished. The message was clear. Mother knew what she was talking about when she said "I'd better be a good boy."

I would lie in bed and wonder what God looked like. I viewed him as a large cumulous cloud with an old man's face. I can remember, at those times, trying to imagine what existed before God created the heavens and earth. I would try to imagine nothing. What would it be like if there were nothing at all in the universe? Would it be dark, a vacuum? That question left me with a sense of a presence that I could not define. It was while in college that the mystery was solved! In a philosophy class we were studying the Cartesian theories, and the light came on in my mind as I read the quote that is the essence of Descartes' works: "I think, therefore, I am." To imagine nothing affirms the presence of an observer. God has always been here.

Development of faith was a growing experience. I sensed that all men had the need of something to fall back on during times of trouble. There were times I really prayed hard. Like when Janie was sick and when Dad was sick and perhaps before a big test in school when my preparation was less than adequate.

But I felt faith was an individual option. I realized there were many churches and different religions, and I felt everyone had to develop his own relationship with God. People would have totally different needs and beliefs. No man could stand alone, and there were times when all of us would ask the Supreme Being for strength and help. I had no quarrel with those who had different beliefs. I believed it was a condition of man that he would have needs and times of weakness and temptation. In those times he would have to rely on support from another source. It was only important that a man believe and have faith in God.

Church slowly became a social experience. As my faith grew, I began to see the benefit of shared faith. This provided an organized support group ready to respond in times of trouble. This support rallied a strong sense of strength that developed endurance, commitment, satisfaction, relief and acceptance during times of trouble.

My attention span in Sunday School was always affected by an eagerness for it to be over so I could play golf, go fishing or go hunting with Dad and Fred. It was difficult for me to apply the lessons of the Scriptures to a 20th century childhood. The lesson that made the greatest impact was reading of the gospel according to Matthew. *"Do unto others as you would have them do unto you."* That seemed to be the answer to all the problems in the world. If I would just treat everyone in the manner I would like to be treated, I would have a good relationship with everyone. I had always assumed that the inverse of that was also applicable. I felt that I could expect to be treated in the manner that I would treat another. Was it too much for me to expect to receive the same level of care that I strive to deliver?

The lessons of judgment and forgiveness were also introduced in Sunday School classes and reinforced at home. The concept to "turn the other cheek" was particularly difficult to understand. If people treated each other in the manner that they wanted to be treated, there would be no need to "turn the other cheek." But one day our teacher told us, "It is easy to love those who befriend you. The real test of a Christian is to love his enemy. We are all God's children and every man is a brother."

"Let he who is without sin cast the first stone." This lesson reminds us that none of us is perfect and that we should not judge our brothers. I have tried to remember these lessons in relating to my fellow man. A review of my chart has really put me to the test. I am in conflict with my duty to God and my oath as a physician. I can forgive the errors as they have affected me personally, but to ignore them might result in a similar outcome to another patient. "The other cheek" might, in effect, be any future patient. As a physician, I cannot overlook the violations of our commitment to the delivery of the best health care possible.

TWENTY-TWO

PoPo always joked that he married my grandmother young so he could raise her the way he wanted. She had a knack of making him feel like he ran the show while she puttered along independently playing her own part as she wished. She was energetic, creative and always in control of every domestic issue. When her eyesight failed, she had no problem sewing, cooking or cleaning house and learned to cope with being blind by trial and error. After I returned from Vietnam, Mary Lynn and I went to her house for fried chicken and all the trimmings, including mashed potatoes and gravy without a lump to be found. I went to the kitchen while she was preparing the meal and asked her how she could have the chicken frying and biscuits in the oven and be stirring the gravy and know when each was done. "Oh, the old stove and I have been around a long time!"

After PoPo died in 1964, MoMo continued to live in Paola. When Mary Lynn and I moved to town, Dad convinced MoMo to move into an apartment in Ottawa. She remained spry and active until she began losing weight in her 90th year. Tests revealed a carcinoma in her stomach. She began to have choking spells and continued her weight loss and wouldn't eat properly. After one severe spell, I hospitalized her. It was apparent that choking, vomiting and aspiration of the emesis were her greatest threats. I told her she was going to have to move to a different apartment where a nurse could call on her, a nice way to say a nursing home. She simply nodded and agreed. Several weeks after the nursing home placement, I got a call from the nurse at 5 a.m.

"Your grandmother had a severe choking spell in the night. She is all right now, but she wanted you to know."

I went to the hospital to make rounds after showering and shaving. On my way out of the hospital, I stopped by the medical records department to dictate some overdue charts. Halfway through the dictation, I suddenly stopped and realized I needed to go see MoMo. The charts would wait.

As I walked into her room, she was lying in bed fully dressed as if she was going somewhere.

"Hello, MoMo, how are you?"

"Hello, Bud, I'm fine. I have had a great life. PoPo is gone. I've watched your family grow. Your folks, you and your family are all I have left."

I checked her stomach and blood pressure, gave her a kiss and said, "I'll see you tomorrow."

I went to see another patient down the hall at the nursing home. As I turned to speak with the patient, the nurse was at the door.

"Your grandmother has passed."

She died as she had lived, without a whimper. After the funeral, I told the minister what a miracle it was that I happened to be moved to stop dictating and go visit MoMo at that time.

"I have a feeling she would have waited for you."

My father married a nurse from a small town in central Missouri. My mother is out of the same mold as my grandmother. Her control of every situation, her dedication to family and her unshakable faith in God have kept her going through an unbelievable series of personal tragedies.

As her first born, I was destined to carry the family banners. I got off to an inauspicious start. I had a personality conflict with my kindergarten teacher. The conflict was that she didn't like me and I didn't like her. The end result was an F the first semester and the boot the first day of the second semester. Mother would not be denied. It was straight to the superintendent of schools! I changed schools and was reinstated as a passing student. Mother was inwardly vindicated when the first teacher ran off with the bus boy from the North American Hotel several weeks later.

My mother stood firm when my sister Janie had polio and endlessly supported her determination to live as normal a life as possible. She would adjust her lip and insist, "It's the Lord's will. Things will work out for the best. Trust the Lord."

High school and college went well for all of us. Fred and I were at the drive-in theater in 1961 when the message came over the speaker.

"Bud Gollier, report to the snack bar. It is urgent!"

I ran down to the concession stand and was told: "Go to the hospital in Ottawa. Your Dad had a heart attack. Don't hurry, he's okay."

I knew then that the message had come from Mother, but I didn't know whether I believed her or not. I called the hospital and she came to the phone and reassured me, but I was not totally convinced all was well. Fred and I raced home, and the first person we saw was Mother, who was just as calm as could be.

Dad recovered well, but the next shock was the most devastating, Janie's Hodgkin's disease. Janie noted a lump in her neck one day, and a biopsy confirmed Dad's fears. In the early 1960s, Hodgkin's disease was not as effectively treated as it is now. Janie continued to act as if nothing was wrong. She became a cheerleader in high school, went to the University of Kansas and joined Kappa Alpha Theta. She was always looking forward to something and always looked at the bright side of things.

I knew the prognosis was not good, but Mom and Dad refused to buckle. They looked at the positive aspects. Dad searched the medical literature desperately looking for some sign of a cure. He read everything he could get his hands on. Finally, his determined rational approach to Janie's illness began to waver. One Saturday evening, while I was in medical school, Dad looked up at me after dinner with the saddest blue eyes I have ever seen.

"Bud, I want you to fly to Montreal next week. There is a clinic there, and they have reported some success in treating Hodgkin's with a new drug made from apricot pits. They call it Laetrile. Most people say it's a quack remedy, but if it turns out to be a cure, I'd never forgive myself. I bought your plane ticket. Here's the name of the clinic and the address."

He handed me a piece of paper with the address of the clinic along with the plane ticket.

"They said they'd save some for us. You'll have to put the

medicine in a suitcase. Don't report it to customs. It's not a controlled substance, but it's not approved for use in the U.S. It's worth a chance." His voice trailed off.

"Oh, Bob, don't sound so bleak," Mom said. "Everything will be okay."

We went to church the next morning. Janie's boyfriend, Tracy Bradford, came for dinner. Tracy was an Ottawa University student who had taken quite a shine to Janie.

As we sat down to dinner, Mom asked Tracy to say the blessing. Tracy was the son of a Baptist minister, and I knew I was in for more than a short verse.

"Dear Heavenly Father, we thank you for this food. Help us to use it to fulfill Thy plans for us. We thank you for our many blessings. We thank you for good friends, good times, the beautiful flowers and the crops in the field."

It was getting darker outside as the clouds were gathering. I looked at Janie. She smiled and rolled her eyes to the ceiling. My stomach growled.

Tracy went on, "We pray for peace in Vietnam and we pray for good health. Finally, dear Lord, we thank you for this beautiful bright spring day."

A flash of lightning lit up the room! The immediate thunder clap indicated the storm was directly above us.

"I think the Lord has just said Amen, Tracy," Janie said, with an embarrassed giggle. "Whee," she said.

"Tracy," said Janie, "I didn't think you'd ever quit!"

"I have a lot to be thankful for."

Tracy and Janie laughed and giggled all through dinner. I let them know I thought they were pretty silly.

After dinner, Tracy excused himself. "My dad is coming down from Omaha this afternoon. I told him I'd meet him in the dorm."

Janie went up to her room. A foreboding silence gripped the room.

"Bob, we've got to tell Tracy."

Mom's voice was firm.

"He probably knows."

"He doesn't act like it."

Dad looked at me. "Buster, I've got one more job for you to do."

"I know."

Tracy's father was a distinguished gentleman with curly gray hair. He was walking to the door of Tracy's room as I entered the dorm. I hailed him and we met at the door as Tracy opened it.

"Bud, what a pleasant surprise!" he said in greeting.

Tracy gestured us in and sat on the laundry hamper as we sat on the bed.

"Did you have a nice trip, Dad?" Tracy said.

"Not too bad. There isn't as much truck traffic on Sundays."

I was uneasy with the small talk. Might as well get it over with.

"I have some bad news," I said, a little too loudly. I swallowed hard and reached for my handkerchief.

"Janie's real sick. She has Hodgkin's disease."

Tracy was solemn.

"There isn't a cure. There's nothing to do."

"We can pray," Rev. Bradford said.

"Tracy, you didn't tell me about this."

"I didn't know for sure. I'd heard the rumors, but Janie never talks about it. She just talks about other things. She never talks about herself."

"Son, you've got your work cut out for you."

I took Mary Lynn to have dinner with my folks and Janie to announce our engagement. I had never seen Janie so happy when we broke the news. Mary Lynn and I had been dating for approximately six months and the romance had grown after an inauspicious beginning. When I met her parents early in our romance, her mother had said, "This will never last! You're both wasting your time. Mary Lynn can't stand doctors!"

****

After dinner, when we announced our intent to marry, Janie looked up and smiled and said, "Well, Bud, it's about time. This has been one of your better days!"

One day in the summer of my junior year of medical school in 1965, Janie developed pneumonia and went into the hospital. I was on a preceptorship in the western part of the state when she took sick.

The first warning of personal tragedy often comes with the piercing ring of a telephone as it shatters the stillness of the night.

"Hello," I mumbled after groping for the phone in the strange bedroom at my preceptor's home.

"Bud," Fred's familiar voice jolted me out of my stuporous state. "Janie just passed away. Mom was with her when she died. She really went downhill in a hurry. The Laetrile didn't work."

"How are Mom and Dad?"

"Doing pretty well. Mom better than Dad as usual. She was ready for it."

"I'm about 200 miles away. I'll grab a quick breakfast and be in Ottawa in four hours."

"Be careful."

"Don't worry."

I had a week to go on my rotation, and I told the preceptor that I had to go home for the funeral and would be back the next day to complete my service. He shook his head and said, "Your work is done here. You must be home with your family."

As I walk into my mother's home now, a picture of my sister sits in her kitchen. Beneath the picture is the verse:

> " 'Twas midnight, not a spoken word.
> Just a moment of emotion —
> A lifetime of deep devotion
> God spoke and she was gone."

One day my mother and I were discussing her family tragedies.

"I have always been distressed when I hear some people bemoan their loss at a funeral with the plea — why me? I don't have a particularly low opinion of myself, but I have never wasted time wondering why all these things were happening. My question is — why not me?"

After that conversation, I began to understand why it took me so long to ask questions about my care.

Some of Mother's good common sense had rubbed off!

After Mary Lynn and I were married, we moved to Phoenix for my internship at Good Samaritan Hospital. Fred was stationed with the Navy in San Diego. He spent nearly every weekend with us. It was necessary on weekends to escape the stifling heat of the valley. We would travel to Sedona or up to Flagstaff and explore Zane Grey's Mogollon Rim Country.

One weekend Fred came over and we decided to go to the White Mountains north of Globe for some trout fishing on the Apache Indian Reservation. On our way out of Globe, up the beautiful Salt River Canyon, we were captured by the beauty of the rushing Salt River as it tumbled down the rocky canyon. As we neared Show Low, the cattle corrals near the highway were all full as they had been herded to pens for pick-up on the way to market.

Fred and I were eagerly anticipating the fishing as Mary Lynn suddenly said, "What are all those cows doing crowded in those pens?"

"That's to protect them from the turkeys," I quickly said.

"The turkeys?"

"Yes, in the White Mountains the turkeys are the main predator to the cattle."

"How big are these turkeys if they attack cattle?"

"Well, last week they found a dead one that weighed 450 pounds. There was a picture of it in the Arizona Republic."

"The turkeys at Thanksgiving and Christmas aren't that big!"

"Those are just the chicks."

Fred couldn't stand it.

"Mary Lynn, you're at a real disadvantage. Bud and I grew up with Dad and PoPo pulling our legs all the time."

"Yes, I remember one time PoPo said he would give me a nickel if I could tell him who was buried in Grant's tomb."

A few miles down the road Mary Lynn said tentatively, "It's Grant, isn't it?"

More than 20 years of a fabulous marriage has been filled with a lifetime of happy times. The years have been sprinkled with our share of disappointments, for sure, but neither of us would trade a day of our time together. I have always believed that, in the union of marriage, the marriage assumes a personality that is a by-product of the two partners. The strength of that marriage is directly related to the effort that each person contributes. Mary Lynn's effort will never be questioned. She has adapted herself in a beautiful manner. She is able to live her life and express her personality, and she makes me think I'm in charge.

Bo Killough, my partner in the farming operation, helped me plan a surprise 40th birthday party for Mary Lynn. We rented the Kiwanis Cabin at Lake Pomona, a reservoir 15 miles west of Ottawa. Bo barbecued a pig. He was afraid of rain, so he hauled in two truckloads of rock so none of the guests would get stuck. Mary Lynn, the kids and I got on our pontoon boat with Mike and Susan Latimer and their boys. Mike shares Mary Lynn's birthday. We told the birthday couple we were going to cook hamburgers on the boat. We motored around, and as the prearranged hour neared, we circled the Kiwanis Cabin. Everyone began to gather at the shore. Mary Lynn saw them and said, "It must be a bunch of moonies. I've heard they are having conventions at different parks."

Then suddenly she turned and said, "Oh, Bud, turn off the motor, they're singing something!"

"Happy birthday to you, happy birthday to you!"

The blank expression on Mary Lynn and Mike's faces exploded into realization as the children handed them their party caps that had a big 40 in bright letters above the bill. Bo Killough put on the perfect party and everyone had a ball!

TWENTY-THREE

I CAN REMEMBER the grim look on my father's face when I was in college and we made the trip to visit my dying grandfather. PoPo looked at me and said, "Bud, if you ever have a patient with cancer of the prostate, cut his head off." I could feel my father wince. As we drove home, he simply said, "I wish there was something I could do." To my children, I was Daddy, so my father was, naturally, Big Daddy, and that was as it should be, for he had pushed 280 pounds most of his life.

When he retired from medical practice because of heart disease, he didn't seem to enjoy fishing as much. When he was working hard, he felt he had earned an afternoon off and fishing was a passion. He then developed a progressive weakness and muscle wasting associated with muscle and bone pain. The most difficult part of his illness was the lack of an exact diagnosis. There was talk of lupus or amyotrophic lateral sclerosis, Lou Gehrig's Disease, but all the tests were inconclusive, and even a trip to the Mayo Clinic failed to solve the dilemma of his progressive weakness and muscle atrophy. The consensus was that he suffered from a neuropathy or degenerative nerve disorder as a result of adult-onset diabetes mellitus. The lack of a diagnosis or, more specifically, a treatment plan that would offer relief or cure, was most frustrating for him. It was ironic that after many years of relieving pain and suffering for his patients, he would have an illness that could not be cured.

His mind remained sharp, and this was perhaps the key to his frustration. He knew what he wanted to do and had goals, but his body failed him. Retirement was a horrible mistake for him. He had lost his sense of purpose and no longer felt he was useful. It is sometimes a blessing when the mind gets old before the body; at least you don't know what you are missing. It is an ideal situation when the mind and body age in concert; then it is easy to grow old gracefully.

Just as Big Daddy had cared for PoPo at the end, proximity and devotion saw to it that I would attend to Big Daddy. He had many episodes of chest pain, and I hospitalized him a number of times for pain relief and adjustment of medication. His heart problem was well documented, and he had had two coronary bypass operations with effective relief of his pain and improvement in his condition each time. However, the muscle wasting and weakness was a separate entity. He had a sense of impending doom and seemed to be more discouraged with each passing week. Antidepressants were of no benefit, and caring for him was terribly frustrating. I couldn't think of anything to do for him, but I was in good company. A host of specialists from Metropolitan Hospital, the Medical Center and the Mayo Clinic had no better idea than I had, but they did not share my empathy with him. He was not their father. They had not seen him down four quail on a covey rise or hit a golf ball 250 yards or catch crappie on ultra-light fishing equipment when they were spawning on the shoreline. They had not seen the gentle care of this loving physician.

Big Daddy had an extraordinary devotion to his profession and to his patients. His success was due to the fact that his patients sensed that devotion.

One Sunday morning, Mother called and said Dad was having the most severe pain he had ever had. I rushed over and gave him a hypo and told Mother to call the ambulance. He stopped her and said, "No, we're not going to the hospital this time."

He looked at me and said, "Bud, I have always told you there is a time to pull the tubes and let a man die with a little dignity."

Mom persisted.

Dad shook his head.

"We have to do something!"

"Not this time, dear. I love you."

Dad's eyes rolled back. I began to compress his chest. Mother called the ambulance. I gave him an ampule of adrenalin in the vein. He did not respond. When the ambulance arrived, I checked his pupils. They were fixed and dilated.

"Mother, this is the time."

"I know," she said softly.

At the funeral, the Reverend Henry Roberts was delivering the eulogy. Henry was a longtime friend and shared Dad's love for the outdoors. We had fished, hunted and played golf together many times.

The packed funeral home was a testimony to the respect the community held for my father. After reviewing the history of his life, Henry digressed into a review of a fishing experience they had shared.

"Bob and I were out on the lake early and the crappie were in the shallow water near the shore. With my rig, I was having trouble casting the small feathered jig. Bob was catching fish, one after the other, and I was having trouble getting my bait in the water. I finally caught a few, using Bob's spare rod.

"After we finished cleaning the fish in his garage, Bob went to his car and got out his favorite ultra-light rod. As he handed it to me, he said, "Henry, I want you to learn to fish for crappie — properly."

And from the Apocrypha and Ecclesiasticus in the New English Bible:

Honour the doctor for his services
For the Lord created him
His skill comes from the Most High,
And he is rewarded by kings.
The doctor's knowledge gives him high standing
And wins him the admiration of the great.
The Lord has created medicines from the earth,
And a sensible man will not disparage them.
Was it not a tree that sweetened water
and so disclosed it properties?
The Lord has imparted knowledge to men,
that by their use of his marvels he may win praise;
by using them the doctor relieves pain

and from them the pharmacist makes up his mixture.
There is no end to the works of the Lord,
Who spreads health over the whole world.
My son, if you have an illness, do not neglect it,
But pray to the Lord, and he will heal you.

BOOK THREE

The Rest of the Story

TWENTY-FOUR

ALTHOUGH I HAVE successfully met many challenges, I have been frustrated in an effort to return to golf as a form of rewarding recreation.

Golf has long been a family interest. Big Daddy was the state Sand Green's Champion in high school. This was due to the a fierce competitive drive and a compact powerful golf swing that he had learned from my grandfather. His success was also due in no small part to his ability to rake a sand green in a manner that could be likened to constructing a trough to the hole.

Fred and I both began our golf careers as Dad's caddies when the main duty was to keep quiet and stay out of the way. We had an assortment of cut-down, wood-shafted clubs during our early years and started swinging at balls whenever we had a chance. PoPo was always encouraging us and would berate Dad for not playing with us as much as he had played with Dad at that age. We would have family games at Paola and Osawatomie, and PoPo would brag to all who would listen about his grandchildren. When the tournaments were played in the summer, PoPo would be in the gallery as Fred and I played ourselves out of contention by some bad bounce or uncommon stroke of horrible luck.

One Sunday at the Paola Invitational, PoPo had outdone himself. We had played with him the day before, and both Fred and I were right around par for the day. PoPo had arranged for us to be paired with two hot-shot Paola youths and was telling one and all that one of us would win the tournament and be the third Gollier champion of the Paola Invitational. Both he and Dad had won the tournament in years past.

We both started poorly, and when we got to the fifth tee, we were both way over par. The fifth hole is a 180-yard par three, and for those with sporting blood, the men's Golfing Association offered a three-to-one bet on hitting a ball onto the green. All four of us put a dollar down and, of course, PoPo put a dollar down on Fred and me. We were all unsuccessful, and my tee shot was just the beginning of disaster for me as I chopped my way to a smooth nine and out of the competition. On the second nine holes I meekly climbed the steps to the fifth tee. PoPo was way in the back of the crowd as a loud-mouthed elderly gentleman shouted, "Gollier, here's your grandson again; get your money out. I betcha $5 none of the four of them hit it onto the green!" Not to be laughed at, we all put our dollars down again. As before, the first two boys missed the green. Then Fred missed slightly to the left. As I teed up the ball, I heard the man say to my grandfather, "I'll let you out of the bet. This boy had a nine last time!"

PoPo winced as I turned to the man and pulled a $5 bill out of my pocket and said, "Cover that if you don't mind, sir!"

I took a five iron and hit the ball right at the flag. It landed two feet from the hole and didn't move an inch. I took the money from the man who was putting up with a lot of chatter from my grandfather and promptly went to the green and missed the putt.

I inherited my father's competitive drive, but one of the main ingredients to his formula for success was eliminated with the transition of most courses in the Middle West from sand to grass greens. I had learned as much as I could from him in the development of the grip and swing and enjoyed modest success in high school. After I settled in Ottawa, I was fortunate enough to be on the winning team in the annual Labor Day tournament, which was the social highlight of the summer, an activity that was enjoyed by all. That success was followed the next year by one of those "every dog has his day" experiences. I was playing in a fund-raising event, which attracted several touring pros to help raise money for charity. As luck would have it, I was paired with Grier Jones, who had enjoyed some success on the pro tour. He was a former All-American golfer from Oklahoma State and was well known in our area. I was nervous as could be when I heard the pairing and was afraid my inconsistent short game, complete with a variety of missed hits, including the bane of all golfers — the shank — would ruin Grier for life. I was so apprehensive I had perfect concentration and swung easily and had excellent tempo all day.

When it was over, I had shot a 70 to Grier's 71. It was the second sub par round I had ever shot. Not bad for a country boy with an eight handicap!

When playing golf after my illness, I could still hit the full shots well enough, but when finesse was called for, my depth perception problem raised its ugly head. I fell to a 22 handicap and the frustration grew. My problem was that I couldn't forget that I had been able to play better. I was unable to be satisfied with average play. I forgot that I was lucky to be able to play at all.

When Bo and John took up the game seriously, I felt I needed to play to share experiences with them. It didn't bother me that they could beat me, but it infuriated me that I was so inconsistent. Others would say I could get it back if I would just work at it, but they didn't understand. With the pitching wedge and short approach shots, I was completely helpless. I either hit way behind the ball, topped it or shanked it straight right. One day when playing with Bo, he said, "Dad, you're playing the ball way too far forward in your stance on your short shots. You need to move it back farther when using the lofted clubs."

I tried his suggestion and was shocked to find he was right.

"I have played this game all my life and had numerous lessons and no one ever told me that!"

As we played the rest of the round and I hit the ball straight at the pins, I was staggered. As we finished and walked off the last green, I looked at Bo.

"That was a good tip you gave me, but a willing student is just as important as an effective teacher."

I then decided to once again play in the Labor Day tournament and had the good fortune to have the Rev. Henry Roberts as my partner.

The second day of the tournament was Sunday, and Henry and I were scheduled to tee off after church. I decided to attend his service that day. As he gave the children's sermon, he asked them if they knew what Labor Day is celebrated for. He then lapsed into a discussion of the work ethic, and he suddenly stopped and looked at me, smiled and said, "Children, anything worth doing is worth doing well."

It was truly a feast or famine round of golf that final day. I had four birdies, two double bogies and an inglorious 10 on the sixth hole. After the sixth hole, instead of hanging my head and sulking, I played the next 12 holes in four over par, and we climbed back to seventh place in the final standings. Not the Penthouse, but not the Outhouse either! It was very rewarding to play a respectable game of golf for the first time in several years.

But success is as fickle in the game of golf as it is in the game of life. The next year disaster struck in the Labor Day tournament. My partner was Charlie Porter, an Ottawa native who remains a longtime friend. Charlie is as competitive as a person can be. His intense concentration is disturbed only by the intermittent plaintive cries of "Oh, Charlie," as his shot falls short of his expectations. Charlie played well both days of the tournament and had only one serious misfortune. He hit a ball into the rough on the fifth hole on the first day, and as he addressed the ball, he moaned. I thought he was in pain. Then he looked up and said, " My dad always said, 'Charlie, if you don't like it in the rough, hit it in the middle.'"

He liked what he said so well, he said it again: "Charlie, if you don't like it in the rough, hit it in the middle." Luckily, I rose to the occasion on that hole and saved our par. After the first day, we were in fifth place, a great position to make a run for the championship on the last day.

I was not up to the challenge. Charlie once again was superb, shooting a two over par 73 to go with his opening round of 70. My respectable opening round, 87, gave me some hope, which was quickly abandoned. The sixth hole was again my downfall. Just as the Augusta National, the site of the Master's, has its Amen Corner, the Ottawa Country Club has its Amen Corner with the fourth, fifth and sixth holes bordered by a treacherous out-of-bounds to the right. Each player is awarded two "mulligans," a chance to replay an errant shot. I used both of my mulligans on number six, the third leg of Amen Corner, reducing a disastrous 10 to a horrible six. Nonetheless, I recovered and finished the front nine with the 42 within sight of my goal of 84. However, I had to play the Amen Corner again on the second nine without mulligans. As I teed it up on number five, Charlie said, "Swing easy and watch the ball!"

I watched it sail out of bounds across the road into the front yard of a farmhouse. I quickly teed up again.

"Take your time," Charlie pleaded.

Out again.

Quickly I hit a third and it sailed into the left rough. There was nothing to say as Charlie and I walked down the road to retrieve my balls.

"Bud, I didn't see whether the second one crossed the road or not. Where did it end up?"

"I couldn't see through the tears," I said.

I struggled to a 12, knowing we were out of the competition. I settled down somewhat and played the last four holes in two over par, sinking a 30-foot putt on the last hole for a birdie two, just like a man who could play the game. We ended up 14 under par and I had a fat 92, which lost five strokes to par after my handicap was subtracted. Had I just shot my handicap, we would have finished in the money. As they posted our score, I remembered a saying I had heard from PoPo years before:

"Every shot makes somebody happy."

Fred and I had been in the gallery in 1960 at Cherry Hills in Denver when two legends collided in the U.S. Open. It was Ben Hogan's last fling at the prize of the U.S. Professional Golf Tour. He was playing with a young amateur who was making his first run at the championship. The young amateur, of course, was Jack Nicklaus, who was just beginning his dominance of professional golf. It was a thrilling match! So thrilling that we were spellbound. Not wanting to miss a thing, we stayed with Hogan and Nicklaus the entire round and missed the main event, as Arnold Palmer was shooting lights out several holes behind us. Fred and I had reminisced about our Cherry Hills experience many times over the years, and Bo and John were well aware of the story.

In the summer of 1985, we had an offer of tickets to a practice round of the P.G.A. Tournament at Cherry Hills. Bo, John and I jumped at the chance. We followed Curtis Strange and Fred Couples for eight holes. Bo wanted to follow one group for the entire round so he would have an opportunity to see the entire course. As we walked from the eighth green to the ninth tee, we noted that a group was just finishing putting on the first green. As we looked up the fairway, Bo exclaimed, "Tom Watson!"

Tom was playing with Hal Sutton and Jim Colbert, and we followed them the entire round. Tom shot a credible 66, and it was a real thrill for Bo to be so close to one of the game's greatest players.

While Bo and I were watching Tom, John was quietly doing his own thing. He had bought a souvenir 18th flag from Cherry Hills and was getting autographs. On the plane home I looked at John's loot. The names on his flag included Hal Sutton, Raymond Floyd, Fuzzy Zoeller, Bernhard Langer, Tom Watson, Hubert Green, Jack Nicklaus and Arnold Palmer.

As we stormed in the house after our flight home, the boys were both talking at the same time telling Mary Lynn about their exciting day. I suddenly realized that the Cherry Hills experience in 1960 was old news and must be relegated to the archives.

A few weeks later, I joined a twosome for a quick nine holes. One of them was Bill Ruff from Billings, Montana, visiting Ottawa on business. Bill seemed to delay a little as he addressed the ball for a 90-yard approach over the lake to the second green. He finally took the club back and then groaned as the shank of the club sent the ball straight right into the lake. He threw another ball down in disgust. Another shank.

"Oh, shit!"

He hit a third. It skipped weakly across the lake. He picked up his clubs and trudged around the lake. By then, the fourth hole, Bill was beside himself.

"This Kansas heat is close. I'm used to low humidity."

"The heat isn't the only thing bothering you, is it, Bill?"

On the next hole I was standing behind Bill as he looked at the green, 90 yards away. He winced and yanked his wedge out of his bag. He addressed the ball, holding his wedge as if he had a hold on a three-foot rattlesnake! I looked at the ball as he began his back swing. Sure enough, the ball was just off his left instep. Sure enough, straight right and out of bounds. As we retrieved his ball, I said, "Bill, we haven't known each other long, but I can't make you any madder than you are. I'm going to tell you what you're doing wrong. I have a little credibility. I happen to be a world-class shanker. I am the best in the world. I've had lessons and shanked my way from coast to coast. It's a great shot to have in your arsenal. You never know when you may have to hit it around a barn. It's also a great shot to get rid of. All you have to do is move the ball back in your stance with the lofted clubs. You'll hit it lower and straighter. My son showed me that last year and it works."

I hadn't seen the boys behind us. They had slept late and had come out to walk the last few holes with me. They were standing in the shade a few yards from us as I was demonstrating the swing to Bill.

"You remembered that lesson pretty well, Dad," Bo said.

"I try to remember every lesson I learn!"

Bill played the rest of the round without a shank. I was playing well, 2 over par the first 16 holes, and hitting the wedge well. On 17, I hit a 40-yard sand wedge over a tree to about eight feet from the hole. As we walked to the green, Bill said quietly, "Doc, don't ever try to sell me a bridge. That line of bull you gave me on number five was about as smooth as I've heard!"

I looked at him and laughed.

TWENTY-FIVE

I EXPECT to be as effective as I can be in my delivery of care, and I expect my profession to aspire to perfection. It is a fact that the human being is a very complex organism, and a host of difficult-to-predict events can occur at any time, but we must be cognizant of Murphy's Law — "If something can go wrong, it will." Although we must aspire to perfection, we must realize that we will not always attain it. The problem is that our patients and our society have come to expect perfection. This has given birth to the specter of malpractice litigation, and this ominous threat now affects the way we all practice medicine. We order too many tests in order to protect ourselves from lawsuits. We have become robots who have ceased to be effective doctors and to exercise to its highest level that quality that is unique to man, the ability to reason and use good judgment. The quality that will save us all is involvement with and concern for our fellow man, and it is this quality that is best illustrated in the primary care physician. These physicians are personally involved in the lives of their patients and practice medicine with standards as high as many specialists because of their involvement with their community and concern for the well-being of their patients.

The concern for malpractice is shaking the very core of the doctor-patient relationship. To many doctors, every patient is seen as a threat or potential adversary rather than a partner in his care. I view myself as a partner in the care of my patients, but I cannot ignore the fact that in the current environment any bad result may threaten my family's future. In a recent conversation with my surgical colleague and a consulting ear, nose and throat specialist, we discussed the effect of the malpractice crisis on attending physicians.

"What do you do about the stress? How do you deal with that?" my surgeon friend quietly said.

"Do the best I can, that's all I can do!"

The ENT man said he knew of a surgical specialist in the city whose malpractice premiums were $90,000 a year.

"He could do as well to buy a liquor store."

"Better," we all agreed.

"He wouldn't have the risk."

I have an opportunity to bare the soul and capture the essence of the physician — to reveal the pressure, the tension, the stress and the commitment. I have had to reconcile the personal conflict that pervades my very soul when I must deal with the knowledge that a different decision or action might have saved a life or not taken one. It is much more real and harder to forget than the countless decisions we all make every day that sometimes have a deadly effect — the decision of which plane to send a loved one on, whether to pass a car on a hill or whether to ride with good old Jim, who has perhaps had a few too many drinks. The difference is subtle, but based on a very basic premise, trust or maybe faith.

I once admitted an elderly man with emphysema because his family reported he would not eat. He was losing weight and was dehydrated. I started intravenous feedings and ordered blood tests, which were inconclusive and gave no indication of the cancer I suspected. He improved slightly, but continued to lose weight and wouldn't eat despite high protein food supplements. One month later his family brought him back to the hospital in acute distress with emphysema.

"He still won't eat," his daughter said "Could it be his medicine?"

The cobwebs began to clear in my tired brain. Lack of appetite is one of the earliest side effects of digitalis.

"Let me check his blood digitalis level."

It was twice normal despite an appropriate dosage schedule and normal kidney function tests. I had an answer for his lack of appetite, an answer that any sophomore medical student would have had a month earlier. It was of little solace that his emphysema was not affected greatly by the toxic level of digitalis. But why had I been so thick-headed?

There are times when physicians are all too human, too tired, too busy. I have been least effective during those times

I have been stressed. At those times my objective has been to finish the day. The objective has superceded the responsibility to do a thorough and professional job. The patient must avoid the overworked physician at all costs. He must at least avoid the physician who perceives himself as overworked. Many, if not most, physicians enjoy the pace of the busy work atmosphere. It goes with the territory and they work effectively at that pace, but when the pace is uninterrupted and steady, the brain gets tired.

The physician must recognize his frailties and avoid the stress as best he can. The simplest way is to be honest with himself and to be open and honest with the patient. Conscience is the mind's automatic quality control device. It is conscience that insists we learn from our experience, and it is conscience that makes sleep difficult after an unanticipated turn of events.

Stress is taking a different direction in American medicine these days. The original contract was between the doctor and the patient. It was simpler then, but economics has introduced the third party. Insurance companies by the hundreds, Medicare, welfare and Health Maintenance Organizations (HMOs) have all spawned the peer review organization (PROs). These reviewers tell us after the fact whether a patient should have been admitted, when he should have been discharged and whether his care was appropriate. I have no quarrel with the review for the sake of quality. We must all welcome any effort to improve our services, but the review of hospital admissions has given third parties the clout to deny payment to hospitals and has added new stresses to the equation. Hospital administrators and boards are now looking at those physicians who are costing them money. It was much simpler when all you had to do was take care of people.

One Father's Day afternoon, I spent two and a half hours in the hospital medical records department dictating letters to our local peer review organization (PRO), to appeal its admission denials in retrospective review of four of my patients, one of whom had been hospitalized 10 months previously. The PRO has the contract to review Medicare and Medicaid hospitalizations in our hospital as the enforcement arm of the

Health Care Financing Administration under the direction of the Department of Health and Human Resources.

As I finished reviewing the charts and dictating my appeals, the anger in me boiled over. I picked up the dictaphone and dictated the following letter intended to be sent to whomever might care:

Dear Senator:

It is critical that you understand the effect the Health Care Financing Administration review decisions have on the quality of medical care in this country.

I have enclosed copies of appeals of review decisions by the PRO affecting me and my patients. The names and numbers have been blacked out to preserve confidentiality.

As a taxpayer, I am concerned about the merits in a bloated bureaucracy of paying these people who compromise the quality of care.

Each of these cases was retrospectively and incompletely reviewed by a person who has a conflict of interest: To find abuses to justify their jobs or the PRO contract.

As a physician, I object strongly to the attempt to limit the services I provide. The senior citizens should be terrified by the change of priorities in our Federal government.

I practice in a community that is designated critically underserved by federal statistics. Physicians in our community are pressed to provide essential care. It goes without saying that we are not looking for an additional work load by hospitalizing patients unnecessarily.

I also do not have time to answer these confounded reviewers, and it particularly angers me when they don't take the time to do a good review and are being paid with my tax dollars. If the government doesn't want to provide decent care for the elderly, just say so, but don't hide behind the bureaucratic hit men. In the first four months of 1986, Medicare reimbursements have fallen short of services provided to the elderly in *our hospital by $160,000. If this continues, it will amount to $500,000 for the year.*

I would like to know how much I am paying for the PRO Corporation to threaten the very existence of our community hospital. You have done one thing right, you have picked on the right people. You are smart enough to know we will not quit. We are committed to providing care, and we will continue to provide the best care we can afford to provide. If you were reviewing defense contractors this carefully, you would have a different problem. They would simply say, "Go elsewhere!"

No, we will keep trying. I realize this represents only my point of view, but the warnings have been sounded by the medical organizations for years. I refuse to alter the standards of care that have been instilled in me. I hope my rural hospital can keep its door open.

Sincerely,
Bud Gollier, M.D.

When finished, my blood pressure was down to normal and I felt much better.

But, how did we get into this mess? Where did we go wrong? What can we do about it?

Part of the answer to the first question came as I looked at the PRO denial letter. As I looked at the left margin, it hit me like a wet towel in the face. All the officers of PRO, except the executive director, had an M.D. after their names. At the bottom of the list was the medical director, again an M.D. What better way to lend credibility to a corporation designated to review physicians.

It suddenly occurred to me that the socioeconomic environment in medicine, associated with the stress of primary care practice, has spawned a new specialty, a means of quasi-retirement. This newest specialist, following recent specialties of Family Practice and Emergency Medicine, is the medical director. The qualifications for membership vary. A postgraduate medical degree, such as M.D. or D.O., is desired. Board certification is preferred, but not essential. Experience is not a requirement. However, the more experienced, the more likely it is that the medical director will have the quality that is the common denominator in the field. The medical director may be tired. Tired of practice, tired of late night calls, tired of hospital political battles, tired of objective decision making, tired of second-guessing himself when patients don't respond as expected, tired of the fear of being sued and tired of unpredictable schedules. He also must be willing to hide behind the corporate shield when hard decisions are to be made.

I presented my thesis one night at a meeting of our office. One of my partners, a general surgeon, suggested another qualification.

"They must have been at least a partial failure in private practice."

"That's not necessarily true," I said. "They just take advantage of the change in medical practice opportunities. Many of them were just in the right place at the right time."

"What opportunities are you talking about?" my surgeon friend asked.

"Every fledgling HMO or other third-party insurer must have a medical director. The review organizations (PROs) must have a medical director, so the primary care physicians will feel they have representation."

"What do the medical directors really do?"

"Very little. They apply the same rigid criteria sets for each case. A patient is no longer a patient, he is now a diagnosis. If he doesn't fit the criteria, the attending physician spends additional time supporting his decision to admit the patient so his hospital will be paid."

"At a rate far below the cost of services rendered."

"Of course. That is the justification for the concept of Diagnosis related groupings (DRGs). They have determined what the average charges have been for each diagnosis in various regions, and that average will be the reimbursement to the hospital for that diagnosis regardless of the length of stay or services rendered. The patient lost his identity as an individual ... with respect to the hospital's reimbursement."

"I hope that's as far as it goes. We have to hope the individual physician will not compromise the quality of care."

"There are bound to be pressures from administrators and hospital boards to limit lengths of stay and ancillary services."

"We have to resist those pressures."

"As long as we can."

"Back to the medical director," the surgeon continued. "He must also recruit lieutenants to journey to the target hospital to perform peer review, again, a euphemism that implies the reviewer has the flexibility to apply individual consideration to each case."

"Where does he find his lieutenants?"

"From the ranks of the physicians who aren't swamped taking care of people. Those who aren't very busy or those who hope to be promoted to be full-time directors."

"If they hope to be promoted, they better stick pretty close to the manual."

"Exactly!"

"There is another characteristic," my friend said. "Many of the directors have an interest in hospital politics or medical society politics and they truly believe they can do the job better than someone else, so they believe they are doing medicine a favor. They believe if they don't fill the position, some government bureaucrat will come in and be a real stick-in-the-mud."

"Yes," I said, "but they simply lend their good names to the same rigid criteria sets and lend a sense of credibility to retrospective review. The scenario painted by the early American Medical Association warning was very accurate. Now that we are having to live with government intervention, it can only get worse unless we can band together and speak out. These admission denials are potentially depriving people of hospital care they badly need."

"The admission is usually approved in retrospective review if the patient dies."

"Isn't that a hell of a note! That proves they were sick enough to be in the hospital."

"I do not need to ask how much these 'specialists' make. I know full well their salaries are healthier than mine. If that weren't true, they would still be doing what I am doing — working for a living!"

"Do you suppose we're the only ones that think that way?"

"No," I said, "but it's easy to knuckle under. That's what really motivates people to apply for medical directorships. They see a good opportunity and a chance to get out of the rat race."

"You mean if you can't beat 'em, join 'em?"

"Sort of like that, but we do have the obligation to let people know what they're about to lose and that the American health care system is the best in the world. We must defend that devotion to care that has been nurtured by so many physicians over the years."

"Before it's gone forever?"

"Right. This business of the Health Care Financing Administration determining whether care is appropriate by retrospective review and trying to fit every patient into a rigid diagnostic criteria set is the foot in the door."

"And with doctors joining them to lend authority to their operation, it's tough to fight. If the medical directors and PROs don't like our attitude, they can do a better job of communicating with us. It would help if their lieutenants called us and asked for additional information before the official denial. Sometimes I agree with them."

"But they expect us to take a half day off and sit around waiting for the review of our patient's charts."

"As if we didn't have anything better to do."

"We've got to get this message out. Maybe an aroused public can influence some congressmen."

"I hope so."

****

Before dinner on Father's Day, John, a high school freshman and honor student, brought me a glass of lemonade on the patio.

"John, what direction is your education taking you?" I asked.

"I don't know, Dad. I'm pretty good in math. I may go into accounting or be a stockbroker or an engineer."

An empty sad feeling hit me deep in the pit of my stomach. John has an opportunity to be a third-generation physician in our community, following his grandfather and me, and I don't have it in me to encourage him to follow my footsteps. The future doesn't look very bright.

John interrupted my feelings of despair.

"I thought about medicine, Dad, but you spent most of the afternoon working on your day off. I heard you talking to Mom about what you did. If you hadn't put those people in the hospital and they had died, wouldn't you have to worry about malpractice?"

"You've got the picture, John. The lawyers would be two deep at my door."

I breathed a deep sigh. I'm there, I thought. I'm tired enough to qualify. With the new specialty looming as such an attractive opportunity and primary care physicians losing their enthusiasm so rapidly, we will soon have a glut in the new specialty and we will have achieved Nirvana. There will be few primary care physicians for all the directors to direct and few hospitals to review.

But I still enjoy my patients and I like the small town life. I'm egotistical enough to believe I do a pretty damned good job. No, I won't bail out, but I'm sure as hell going to speak my piece. I hope my colleagues will let me join the fight. I haven't had the vision many of them had in the early years. However, the picture is now crystal clear. We have to get involved in our medical association programs or we go down together.

Next, I received a notice from the medical records department informing me they were required to make copies of the charts on all my hospitalizations because I had more denials than the PRO allows. They didn't mention that most of the denials had been reversed on review.

This is the last straw, I thought, as I dictated another fruitless letter.

Dear Medical Director:

I surrender!! You win!! By requesting our hospital to copy all my charts for review because of "too many denials," you have increased the administrative costs and my frustration level to the point that I fully in-

tend to limit my Medicare practice.

I hope a copy of this letter will be of some benefit to me in court if I am sued for "denying" appropriate care and hospitalization to a Medicare patient.

Sincerely, Bud Gollier, M.D.

I once again mailed copies to my representatives in Congress who have shifted their priorities from service and quality of life to spending cuts and budget deficit reduction. I have yet to hear from them.

TWENTY-SIX

IN A RECENT Ann Lander's column, dedicated to the problem of quality medical care, a hospital administrator wrote, "Never mind about back rubs. These days a patient can hemorrhage unnoticed in a $575-a-day room. Nurses must band together and demand quality care for their patients."

Don't lay it all on the nurses. Quality medical care depends on an effective team approach involving nurses, doctors, all support personnel and administrators. Mary Lynn has felt the ineffective care I received resulted from being unlucky enough to get sick on a weekend. It is possible that the administrator at Metropolitan was cutting back on staffing for the weekend and the nurses were swamped. I reported the lack of nurses' notes to Dr. Ford one day. His response was that the blood pressure had to have been taken at the change of shifts and the nurses had to have made notes that had not been recorded on the chart because of the extreme emergency. I simply told him that the evidence did not support that assumption.

After reading Ann Lander's column, my mother tried to placate me by saying, "This sort of thing happens everywhere." A colleague of mine, after reviewing my chart said, "You were just a victim of the system, no one wanted to take charge." That doesn't make it right. I have considered discussing my case with the administrator at Metro, but if my mother is right, the audience is too narrow. My hope is for patients in all institutions to benefit from my experience.

Doctors must learn that nurses are partners and provide an extension of their care. They must give nurses the credit for the great job they do. I have found nurses often make keen observations and it is foolish not to respond to them. I have known some doctors to complain about aggressive and overbearing nurses who "think they're doctors." Perhaps the reason I have no problem with them is I respect them and let them know it. The overbearing nurses may simply be frustrated because they are not being heard. Most nurses are every bit as dedicated as doctors. There are many sacrifices made to complete nurses' training, and they are just as dedicated to quality care as the best physicians.

Recently I had weekend call. A patient, Mrs. Swanson, was admitted late Friday night with a high fever and a urinary tract infection. She was initially started on intravenous fluids and antibiotics. Early Saturday morning I was called to the emergency room to attend a man critically injured in a car accident. It was apparent he needed the care of a neurosurgeon and would have to be transferred 50 miles to the University Medical Center. Because of his injuries and the need to assist with his respirations, I rode in the ambulance with him and was gone for two hours while my partner covered my call.

When I returned, I noted Mrs. Swanson seemed more lethargic and tests revealed she was diabetic as well. I added insulin to her IV and took the beeper to Sara Jane's basketball game. Thirty minutes later, I was called by nurse Vicky Fowler, who reported Mrs. Swanson was less responsive and her blood pressure had dropped slightly. I went to the hospital and increased the intravenous fluid rate. Fifteen minutes later Vicky called again and said the pressure had dropped another 20 points. I had her insert a urinary catheter and measure the urine output hourly to determine whether circulation to the vital organs was adequate. She called again in 20 minutes and said there was no urine in her bladder and that the increased fluid rate had not increased her blood pressure. I raced to the hospital, and we immediately transferred Mrs. Swanson to the Intensive Care Unit. She was obviously developing shock as a result of the bacteria entering her blood system. She needed aggressive support while the antibiotics did their job. We added a blood pressure elevating medication into the intravenous fluid and put her on a monitor. Her blood pressure responded to the medication and this was reflected by an increase in her urine output. She became much more responsive.

The next day she was free of fever with a normal blood pressure and was normally alert.

As I went into the nurses' station after leaving the Intensive Care Unit, I saw Vicky and the aide who had cared for Mrs. Swanson the afternoon before. I smiled and said, "Nice work yesterday; if you hadn't noted her blood pressure falling, she might not be here today."

We must learn to listen to the nurses. Hospital administrators must learn that there are limits to cost cutting. In many hospitals, weekends are commonly staffed by nurses working 12-hour shifts rather than standard 8-hour shifts. Staffs are often reduced in numbers as well because hospital censuses are commonly reduced for the weekend.

Since the weekend is the time most people would like to be off, weekend duty is often viewed as a hardship and the staff morale is low. The pace of work is also affected. Ancillary services, such as X-ray and lab, as well as physical therapy, occupational therapy and respiratory therapy are restricted to little more than emergency services. Nobody is supposed to be sick on the weekend.

Kent Granger, my lawyer friend, compared my care to the situation he ran into when representing the victims of the disaster when skywalks of the Hyatt Regency Hotel collapsed in Kansas City several years ago.

"One hundred fourteen people were killed and scores were injured. Nobody took responsibility for the structural design. Everyone was pointing fingers. The architect blamed the engineers, the engineers blamed the steel fabricators. They all wanted to pass the buck. I can see the same thing happens in medicine.

"The structural engineers finally admitted they never checked the integrity of the steel connections holding the skywalks to the wall. They claimed it was the responsibility of the steel fabricators to make sure the connections would hold. The administrative law judge found the structural engineers guilty of 'gross negligence, misconduct and unprofessional conduct.'

"As a result of the tragedy, the American Society of Civil Engineers made a policy that would have held the structural engineers responsible. That policy has become the standard of care for civil engineers."

I looked at Kent and said, "What happened to me was not the norm. The patient is on the service of the admitting physician, and he is the one that the consultants respond to. He is in charge. My case was just one of those unfortunate slip-ups."

"So was the Hyatt," Kent responded.

TWENTY-SEVEN

THERE ARE MANY TIMES a physician stands alone. He must succeed or fail based on the decisions he makes. Wrong turns happen all the time. It is easy to develop tunnel vision and cruise down the wrong path reassured by familiar signs and responses on the way to the anticipated conclusion.

I had a patient in the hospital with congestive heart failure. She responded well to diuretics to remove the fluid and to digitalis to strengthen her heart. Her blood tests proved she had not had a heart attack when she came into the hospital. After a few days she was responding well and moved out of the ICU. She then developed a burning pain and nausea. She had a history of ulcers, so I ordered a chest X-ray and an X-ray of her stomach. These were normal, but the burning and nausea persisted. I ordered blood tests to see whether she had too much digitalis in her system, but these too were normal. Her nausea continued, and I gave her medicine to combat it and to block the hydrochloric acid production by the stomach. She seemed to improve and then had another bout of nausea and "burning" in her stomach. I ordered more tests, thinking perhaps she had a toxic level of the medication for her breathing problem. I left the hospital thinking I had done everything. When I got to my office, the call from the nurse came stating the patient had stopped breathing and was unresponsive. A nurse and two doctors were trying to resuscitate her. I rushed back, and after 15 minutes of unsuccessful resuscitations she was pronounced dead of an acute heart attack. As I tiredly drove back to the office, I was thinking how relaxing it would be to be a clerk or deal with paper problems and simple tasks that can be corrected with an eraser. The life of a physician can be very lonely. We are really in trouble when we stop second-guessing ourselves and reviewing our experiences.

A 70-year-old woman was recently seen in the emergency room of our hospital by our emergency room physician, a resident physician from the Medical Center. The patient complained of chest pain, which was relieved by Nitroglycerin, and an electrocardiogram was interpreted by the resident as normal. The patient was reassured and dismissed from the emergency room. Several hours later she had recurrent chest pain unrelieved by Nitroglycerin and was rushed by ambulance to the city where she had an acute myocardial infarction. The dye studies of her coronary arteries indicated she had delayed too long for balloon angioplasty or enzyme infusions to reverse the heart attack. Her course was uneventful and the outcome was satisfactory.

However, the family was very upset that the presenting complaint had been treated so lightly. "She might have died," the daughter implored. I could understand her anger. Her father had been a well-known physician in a neighboring town. I could relate to her concern that her mother deserved better care. I reviewed the emergency room record at her request in my capacity as chief of medicine. The resident had indicated she had a history of stable angina, but this attack had occurred at rest, and even though it was relieved by Nitroglycerin, it was new angina and, by definition, unstable angina. The EKG did reveal some borderline changes that might represent a variation of normal or might represent a clue to an evolving problem. Time solved the mystery, and the result was not catastrophic. There is no question in my mind that I would have admitted that patient. I discussed the case with the resident, and he agreed with my review. The pain had occurred while the patient was attending a graduation ceremony, and her weekend plans included several more commencement activities at her alma mater. She was looking forward to renewing friendships with classmates from years gone by. It is likely she was minimizing her complaints so her weekend wouldn't be spoiled by hospitalization. Perhaps that explains why the resident didn't identify the pain as unstable angina. The resident and I agreed there was a good lesson in this case; attention to a good medical history is critical to our performance as physicians.

I reported the meeting to the patient's daughter, and she was quite satisfied that we had reviewed the case and that some good would come of the experience.

At our medical staff meeting, the audit committee reported that they had reviewed the chart and had concluded that 90 percent of them would have handled the case in the same manner. I told them of my review and my quarrel with their conclusion. "I guess I am in the other 10 percent," I remarked. I suggested that it would be appropriate for the emergency room physician to consult the attending physician on all cases presenting chest pain. That raised a storm of protests. All agreed that this particular case was a tough call. I told them I likely admitted too many people with chest pain, but I could accept being accused of admitting too many people if it would prevent a possible disaster. One of the younger staff members raised his voice and yelled, "Don't you know hindsight is 20/20, Bud? Don't you ever make a mistake?" The anger in me boiled over as I shot back, "I know a little about mistakes, but I have never made one I didn't learn something from."

One evening I had a phone call from a high school friend who said his mother-in-law was having a terrible headache. She had recently been in a hospital with high blood pressure and had been on medication at home. I met her at the emergency room, and her blood pressure was 260/116. She was nauseated and had blurred vision. I admitted her to the ICU, started an IV and gave her a strong diuretic by vein. The nurse rushed up to me while I was writing up her chart and said, "Blood pressure is 290/140!"

"Let's mix up the Nitro-Prusside. We've got to get it down!"

Eight minutes after the Nitro-Prusside drip began, the nurse called out, "Come over here quick!" The patient was moist, but had good color. She smiled and said, "Gee, I feel better."

The nurse looked up and said, "Her blood pressure is 120/70. You sure work fast."

The patient said, "That is wonderful medicine."

I looked at them and said, "Even a blind squirrel finds the acorn once in a while!"

Practicing in a small town has many rewards. The visibility of the small-town doctor is a drawback. The newspaper is your scorecard. Hospital news is reported daily — admissions, births, deaths. The failures are so personal. It can be hell to take care of your friends. If a patient dies, there is a professional sense of failure, coupled with a personal loss and a sense of grief.

Paul Simpson was a good friend. When Dr. David Laury retired, Paul asked me to look after him. He had chronic kidney disease and high blood pressure, a bad combination, but Paul did not complain. He took his medicine and periodically had his blood pressure checked. He was semi-retired and spent as much time as he could with his family. He had a pleasant smile and a friendly word for all he met.

One night, Paul called to say he was having severe upper abdominal pains and bloating after a dinner of chicken-fried steak. He went to the hospital emergency room. I was worried about a heart attack. His EKG was normal and an X-ray of his chest and stomach was normal. His blood pressure was high, 200/120, but he was in a lot of pain. He had a lot of tenderness over his gallbladder. I admitted him to the ICU, still worried about a heart attack. I gave him a hypo for his pain and finally lowered his blood pressure with IV medication. I knew Paul would be a high risk surgical patient if he had a "hot gallbladder," but I didn't feel it was safe to transfer him if he was developing a heart attack. Blood tests would prove whether his heart was responsible for his distress. Our surgeon saw him in consultation and agreed he had an acute abdomen. He felt we should order a gallbladder sonogram to see whether he had stones. Paul was really miserable. The hypos helped ease the pain, but the pain and anxiety were compromising his blood pressure. The sonogram confirmed he had a stone in his gallbladder. The blood test for heart enzyme levels was normal, proving he had no heart damage. I told him we would take his gallbladder out the next day.

"Bud, can't we get it out sooner than that? I can't take much more of this!"

"Let me talk to the surgeon."

The surgeon agreed we could schedule Paul as an emergency at the end of the day. We felt his blood pressure would be easier to control once he was more comfortable. As we wheeled Paul into the operating room, he looked up at me.

"Bud, if you find something else, like cancer, tell the kids. Don't tell their mother."

It was like Paul to think of others at that time. His wife had had some medical problems and he didn't want her to have to worry about him. He wanted me to promise him I would tell his children first and let them tell their mother.

The surgery went well, but his blood pressure was high the entire time. I was anxious to get him into the recovery room so I could monitor his blood pressure and give Nitro-Prusside if necessary. During recovery his blood pressure hovered around 170/100. His pulse was fast, but it was regular. He responded normally and pointed to the endotracheal tube in his throat as if he wanted to say something. He was breathing well and his color was good. We placed Paul in the ICU after the surgery to ensure he would have close observation. The endotracheal tube was removed and Paul continued to be stable. I went home to eat a late supper. As I walked in the back door, Mary Lynn handed me the phone.

"Hello."

"Mr. Simpson's heart just stopped!"

"Oh, shit! Start the resuscitation!"

"We have."

"I'll be right there!"

I raced back to the hospital. A team of nurses and one of my partners were frantically involved in cardiopulmonary resuscitation. Paul had been given Atropine, adrenalin and sodium bicarbonate. We worked for 20 to 30 minutes continuing the cardiac compression and ventilation. The adrenalin and bicarbonate was repeated at regular intervals, but still no blood pressure or palpable pulse.

"It must have been a massive heart attack immediately after the tube was removed."

My partner's voice seemed distant as I was praying I could feel a carotid pulse.

"I guess so," I said weakly.

"His pupils are dilated and fixed," the anesthetist said.

"Son-of-a-bitch," I muttered.

"What went wrong?" said the voice inside me. "His cardiac enzymes were normal. He had a gallstone. He was in severe pain. The pain was making his blood pressure worse," I reasoned.

"Yeah, but he died," the voice said again. "You should have transferred him to the city by helicopter!"

"He was too sick to transfer. He had an acute abdomen."

"He's sicker now." The voice would not be quiet.

I told Paul's family as plainly as I could.

"We could have waited. Maybe it would have quieted down."

"But he was in such pain," his daughter said. "He wanted it out."

"We thought it was the thing to do. I'm so sorry."

"You did your best, Doctor. Thank you."

Sleep did not come easily that night. I tossed and turned. The little voice would not leave me alone.

"You should have waited. What did you miss?"

At 3 a.m. I got up and slipped on my clothes.

"Where are you going?" Mary Lynn asked. She knew I wasn't sleeping well and she roused easily.

"I'm going out to the hospital to look at Paul's chart. Maybe I missed something."

"In the middle of the night?"

"It's the least I can do."

I drove the eight blocks quickly. The nurse in ICU handed me the chart. The blood tests were all normal. The EKG was normal. His kidney function test was high, but that shouldn't have had any effect. The potassium was normal. The blood pressure was the culprit! It was too high.

"You shouldn't have operated on him. He was in no shape for the anesthesia," the voice would not be quiet.

"I know," I muttered. "I thought his pain was making his blood pressure worse. His gallbladder might have ruptured."

"But it didn't!"

"I know it, damn it!"

The nurse was looking at me strangely. I smiled at her and said quietly, "Just having a little conversation with my conscience."

I drove home silently. The little voice was quiet.

Mary Lynn was awake. She had brought me a fresh glass of water.

"What did you find?"

"Nothing. It was just a screwy case."

"Those things happen. You can't be right all the time."

"My patients pay me to be right."

"But you aren't God."

"I know it. But I need to be certain that I learn from every experience. Each case I have had adds to the sum total of my knowledge and will influence my clinical judgment in the future. That's why they call it the practice of medicine."

"You need to do a better job of living with your disappointments."

"Learning from them is a positive way of living with them."

"But they don't seem to get easier to live with as the years go by."

"Arnold Palmer once said when he was young it was easier to forget a bad shot in golf. He would just hitch up his pants and go after the ball and hit it again, knowing he would hit it right the next time. When he got older, he found it took him four or five holes to forget a bad shot. He said he started thinking to himself, 'Arnie, you're a pro. You know better than to play like that. You shouldn't make those silly mistakes.' Mary Lynn, now I know what he meant. When I was younger I would study each case, remember it and look forward to the next challenge, knowing I would do better. But, after 20 years in this business, I look at myself when a patient dies and say, I should have known better. I should have gone the other way. I've been around too long to miss that."

"You've got to quit thinking you always have to be right."

"No, that's where you're wrong. I must always expect to be right. I must accept it when I fall short, but I don't have to like it."

"You're too hard on yourself."

"Tell that to Paul's family."

TWENTY-EIGHT

A YOUNG GIRL, an honor student and cheerleader, was recently killed in our community when she attended a party given by some young adults to celebrate the occasion of a friend's going to court on a DWI charge. Beer and hard liquor were available at the party and provided by the adults. The young girl was lying on a porch railing and seemed to be falling asleep when a young man noted her drowsiness and picked her up to carry her inside. He suddenly lost his balance and fell over the porch railing, and the young girl struck her head on a concrete step as she fell underneath him. She had a massive intracranial hemorrhage and a skull fracture and died instantly. At her funeral, attended by hundreds of her school mates, the minister prayed that authorities would deal with those responsible for this tragedy with a heavy hand. I was surprised and pleased with his strong statement about the folly of providing alcohol to minors and stressing the lesson that we must all learn to be responsible for our actions. As I walked out of the service with Mary Lynn, I asked her about forgiveness. It seemed to me that the minister was violating our scriptural instructions.

One day I saw the minister and asked him about his remarks and about forgiveness. His response did not surprise me. "I am struggling with that," he said. He went on to say that it is critical that all those young people learn a lesson from this tragedy. "Growing and maturing is an evolutionary process. Christianity has evolved from the Old Testament theology to the New Testament theology. We must all continually learn from our experience and grow as human beings as well as Christians."

In telling my story, I have had difficulty reconciling my duties as a Christian and my duties as a physician. In his sixth chapter, Matthew points out that forgiveness is essential. In the fifth chapter, Matthew says, "But now I tell you, do not take revenge on someone who wrongs you." Luke says, "Do not judge others, and God will not judge you; do not condemn them and God will not condemn you; forgive others, and God will forgive you ... The measures you use for others are the ones that God will use for you."

I have no problems with judgment. The standards I have used are the same that I apply to myself. I continually re-examine myself and strive to learn from my experiences. I have no problems with forgiveness. As a Christian, I forgive the doctors and nurses. I am very thankful for my blessings, and as a Christian I can easily "turn the other cheek." As a physician, I have a conflict. I must strive for better care. I owe that to my fellow man. I cannot forgive the failure to meet that obligation or the failure to examine themselves. But how do I reconcile my duties as a physician with my Christian obligations? Is there an element of retribution in my narrative?

As I was researching my moral conflict, I was sitting in the living room watching Syracuse play Villanova in the Big East basketball tournament, and Villanova was winning handily as Syracuse's star, Dewayne "Pearl" Washington, was having an off day. During half-time, I picked up the Bible beside my chair and aimlessly opened it. I was startled to see a bright yellow light circling a passage I had never seen, "No pupil is greater than his teacher; but every pupil, when he has completed his training, will be like his teacher." I wondered where I was and looked at the top of the page, the sixth chapter of Luke. It is appropriate that my dilemma be solved by a physician.

Having been on the receiving end of critical care, I have a unique perspective. A new dimension has been added to my training. In the medical profession, our training must never be considered complete. One of my colleagues recently told me that he felt humbled several times every week. He had practiced medicine for more than 40 years and he still recognizes his shortcomings and continues to re-evaluate himself. So must we continue our training. The responsibility to learn from our experiences could not be stated more clearly than it is stated in the sixth chapter of Luke.

As I looked back down at the Sixth Chapter, the bright yellow circle was no longer there.

****

Orlis Cox didn't look well when he walked into my office. He always seemed indestructible, a living testimony to physical conditioning. His steps were a little shorter and his pace was measurably slower as he walked down the hall.

His shoulders, once broad, rolled forward as he struggled to find a comfortable position in the chair. He seemed confused, as if he was trying to remember why he had come. He suddenly looked 87 years old. His voice quivered as he began.

"Bud, I can't eat anything. No appetite. I seem to be getting weaker. I don't have any energy and I'm losing weight. It's been about six months."

"It doesn't sound good, Mr. Cox," I said. Then I added quickly, "Maybe it's an ulcer. Let me examine you. Have you been having any pain?" I hoped he'd say yes. "No, no pain."

I did a physical exam and included a test of his stool for blood. Everything seemed normal, but Orlis and I knew he was in trouble, big trouble.

"Mr. Cox, you need some blood tests and some X-rays. We'll do them at the hospital in the morning." He didn't bat an eye, but quickly said, "What time?"

"Seven o'clock."

"I'll be there."

The radiologist frowned as he looked at the films. "Looks like a carcinoma of the esophagus. How long has had the symptoms?"

"About six months. He just told me about them yesterday."

"How are the blood tests?"

"We just drew the profile this morning."

"He has a little fluid in his left costophrenic angle," he said as he looked at the chest X-ray. "He may have a pulmonary or lymph node metastasis."

I took a deep breath. "He needs to be scoped for a biopsy. If it's an adenocarcinoma, it might respond to radiation or chemotherapy. If it's a squamous cell, surgery is the only answer and not a good one."

I spoke with Orlis and his wife. "Orlis, you have a growth in your gullet. You'll have to go the Medical Center at K.U. They'll need to look at it with a scope."

"Is it cancer, Bud?"

I looked him in the eye. "We have to prepare for the worst, but hope for the best. They will have to do a biopsy to be certain. I paused and then said, "I'll make the arrangements and we'll visit tomorrow after I get the blood test results from the laboratory. I patted him on the shoulder. He tried to smile and said, "Thank you, doctor."

The blood tests were all normal. There was no evidence of liver or kidney involvement. "The blood tests look good," I said as I walked into the examining room to speak with Orlis and his wife. "I've made arrangements for you to be admitted to the hospital at the Med Center this afternoon."

"You don't waste any time."

"There's no sense stewing about it. It won't go away until we know how to attack it."

"What will they do?"

"The doctor said they would schedule a CAT scan, sort of a three-dimensional X-ray, this afternoon. Tomorrow they will pass a scope into the esophagus and take a biopsy so we'll know what we're dealing with. He said they'd keep you informed and would call me as soon as they had some news."

I didn't hear anything for a few days. When the doctor called, he told me they had had a struggle making the correct diagnosis. "Mr. Cox is an interesting case. When we passed the scope, everything was normal, but the CAT scan revealed a growth wrapped around the lower third of the esophagus. We took some fluid off the chest to look for malignant cells, but the pathologist couldn't see a thing. We tried to do a needle biopsy of the mass, but it was normal. Finally, we had to do an open biopsy. I just got the diagnosis. It is a type of lymphoma that should respond to cobalt therapy. All the residents and interns up here are really excited about this interesting case."

I couldn't wait to interrupt him. "Tell your residents that they're not taking care of an interesting case. They're taking care of a ball park. Our youth baseball park is called Orlis

Cox Field." I then told him about the 1933 National High School Track Championship.

"Oh, my. I see what you mean. We'll take good care of him."

The cobalt therapy was a trial for Mr. Cox. He had a lot of esophageal irritation and wasn't able to take adequate nourishment. Finally, after three-quarters of the therapy, he convinced the doctors he needed a rest and asked to go home to build up his strength before he finished. The doctors called and asked me to follow him at home. They stressed that hope for cure depended on finishing the treatment.

Orlis slowly regained some of his strength, but he had to force himself to eat. I placed him on a high protein liquid diet to build his strength.

One Saturday I stopped by his home on the outskirts of town. He didn't look good. His eyes had lost the twinkle that had always been there due to his eternal optimism and enthusiasm for the task at hand.

"How do you feel, Mr. Cox?"

"Not bad," he answered in a flat voice.

"Are you taking the liquid nourishment?"

"All I can."

"Are you feeling any stronger?"

"Not really."

"How much exercise are you getting?"

"Not much."

I scooted my chair closer to his. "Mr. Cox, I want you to sit up and listen closely."

His eyes showed a hint of the old sparkle as he gathered himself and sat up a little straighter.

"A great man once told me that laziness would beget laziness. I want you to put yourself on an exercise program and walk a mile in 30 minutes twice a day as long as the weather holds. I'll be back next Saturday to see how you're doing."

He tried to smile. "I'll do my best."

"I know you will."

I bid Orlis and his wife good-bye. On the way to the car I found myself hoping it would work. He must finish the treatments. He began to regain some strength.

One day Mrs. Cox called to say he was ready to finish the therapy as an outpatient. I made the arrangements and he made the trip to Kansas City twice a week until his total course was completed. He once again had problems with strength and nourishment.

One afternoon I stopped to see him and he complained of dizziness. His blood pressure was low and dropped significantly when he stood. His mucous membranes were dry, and he had fluid on his lungs.

"Mr. Cox, I have to take you to the hospital. You need some intravenous fluid to treat your dehydration and I'll need to take some fluid off your chest with a needle."

"Okay, let's go."

The hospital course was a struggle for Orlis and his family. I took 500 cc of fluid off his chest and corrected his intravenous fluid deficit, but he continued to deteriorate. I tried to say something encouraging each time I saw him, but I sensed he knew I was just as discouraged as he was.

After a week in the hospital, I told him I needed to remove the chest fluid one more time and would use a larger needle to remove more fluid. I removed nearly a liter of fluid and increased the intravenous fluid rate to guard against hypotension and shock.

He was in the ICU because of an irregular heartbeat and the need for medication to support his blood pressure. After I removed the fluid, his wife and daughters asked that we not use a respirator or life-support if it came to that.

"Daddy's just so tired," they said. Initially he seemed to rest comfortably. He suddenly was restless. His chest was clear, blood gases were normal. His wife and daughters were at his bedside.

He looked at them plaintively, "Can I go?"

Their voices all came together.

"Yes, Daddy,"

And he closed his eyes. Orlis Cox had hit the wall.

TWENTY-NINE

Mary Lynn AND I entered John Peterson's split-level home in the residential area west of the Kansas University campus in Lawrence at 10 a.m. on the Saturday before the big basketball game between the nationally ranked Jayhawks and arch-rival, Kansas State. A win by the Jayhawks would clinch the Big-Eight basketball championship, and there was a feeling of electricity in the air.

John met us at the door and was an imposing sight as his lanky frame was now topped by a thatch of gray, which dominated his once jet-black head of hair. He wore a three-quarter gray beard, which hid the prominent jowl that had been such a characteristic part of his countenance in the past.

"The beard and graying hair don't fool me for a moment, Hoss," I said in greeting.

"Makes me look more like professor, don't you think?"

John was on the faculty in the school of journalism, but 25 years previously, he had been my fraternity brother and teammate on the K.U. freshman basketball team, and after we found that we were not made of the same stuff that sustains traditions, we retreated to interfraternity wars. "Hoss," as he had been known because of his gangly physique and moves similar to a newly born colt, had reviewed an early manuscript of my story, and with his fourteen- year old dog, Ralphey, snoozing on the sofa, we sat down to visit.

"What are you trying to say? What's your theme?" John said as he stomped out one cigarette and lit another.

"A profession's obligation to learn and to strive to improve itself," I offered for starters.

"Yeah, I know, but is your story about your recovery or the hospital stuff?"

"It's not recovery per se. Everyone has a recovery story. Human beings have a lot of resilience, and it's not negligence or malpractice."

"What do you mean?"

"What happened to me was an uncommon event, like the space shuttle disaster. Conditions were ripe for a disaster. The shuttle took off on a cold morning and I got sick on the weekend."

"Don't minimize what happened to you. In spite of what you say, you did have an unusual recovery, and most people don't recover from that serious an illness. I think your ability to come back from that illness is a remarkable feat."

"I didn't have a lot of choices."

"What do you mean?"

"I was just like a twig in a current of water. I just went where the forces compelled me to go."

"What forces?"

"Family, friends, conscience and faith. The story is about family and community support in the throes of calamity."

"With religion as the glue?"

"That's right. One of my first memories of consciousness in that hospital is of a Presence or a Force in my bed lifting me. That feeling was more apparent when Mary Lynn was in my room."

"You've got some good stuff here. Some good sub themes, but why are you telling the story? You say it was an uncommon occurrence, an accident. Why tell the story? I sense a lot of anger in the last part of your story. What are you mad about?"

It came to me all at once — "Duty!"

Ralphey barked and ran to the door. Hoss followed and let him out.

"Damn dog. Had a hell of a time when we sailed to Hawaii, just the two of us. What do you mean — duty?"

"Professional responsibility. I was part of the brotherhood. There have been four great associations in my life: family, fraternity, church and profession. The common denominators in each of those associations were trust, reliance on one another and concern for one another."

"The influence of family and church is very clear in your story."

"In the fraternity house we lea⌐ ⌐ed to rely on one another when we had problems."

"Yeah, I know all about that. I took advantage of that support when my firm went bankrupt on Wall Street. Two of our fraternity brothers, Neil McCoy and Dick Endacott, both crack lawyers, came to New York and saved my ass."

"The next great association I had was with the docs at Metro. I learned a lot from them, and I know they thought a lot of me. When I left for Vietnam, Matthew Drake asked me what I was going to do when I got out of the service. When I told him I was going to Ottawa to practice with Dad, he told me I wasn't setting my sights high enough.

"He said, 'You should finish your residency at the Mayo Clinic. I have some influence there and I'll be glad to write a letter for you.'

" 'Thanks a lot, but I have made up my mind,' " I said to him. Hoss got up to let Ralphey in.

"Let's get back to duty."

"I learned in the fraternity to depend on the brothers. I knew they would stand up for me and they knew I would be there for them. I thought I had the same relationship with the docs at Metro."

"Now you have learned the difference."

"I went down and nobody gave a shit except my wife, my family and the community."

Mary Lynn had been quietly sitting next to Ralphey on the sofa. She sat up quickly. "Oh, Bud, that's not true. The whole hospital was worried about you. They were all just sick."

Hoss interjected, "It's been a long time. You're back to practicing full-time with minimal disability. What have you got to bitch about?"

"Nobody wanted to learn anything.. There is no evidence that anyone ever looked at my chart."

"Bullshit. Some of them were covering their asses, and most of the docs don't even know what happened."

"Bullshit, yourself. They all know. You forget I trained there. They were all good docs in a good hospital. They have the same standards I have. They created me. They know what happened. That's why they were so upset."

"Didn't anyone ever give you a hint?"

"Oh, as I think back on it, maybe that's what the kidney specialist meant when he told Mary Lynn I wasn't ready to hear about my case yet, and maybe Dr. Drake just before he died. One day after I was back in practice, I called him to discuss a pituitary problem. As we finished our visit, he paused and his voice took a strange tone, almost as if it broke. He paused and said, 'Boy, you're lucky to be alive!' "

"But they couldn't say anything, Bud," Mary Lynn interjected. "What would you have them do? Tell you to file a suit?"

"I just expect them to tell me the truth and to indicate they learned something from my experience. No, the statute of limitations took care of the lawsuit. It doesn't protect a person whose reasoning is affected by a cerebral hemorrhage."

"But you say your reasoning was back to normal within six months!"

"Then it was clouded by blind trust. They should have been up front about things. I don't treat people that way and don't hold with people who do."

THIRTY

THE TRIALS and patience of Job have been referred to many times. In studying the book of Job, I have recognized that Job was blessed because of his faith and unwavering belief in God as the Master and Creator. His faith did not waver despite a tragic series of personal setbacks. However, I have questioned the meaning of Job's restoration. After being confronted by God, Job acknowledged God as wise and great and repented all the wild and angry words he had used. Job was restored to his former condition with even greater prosperity. The Lord gave Job twice as much as he had before. The Lord blessed the last part of Job's life more than the first. I had still been unable to forget Job's terrible personal losses. It was hard for me to understand how one could be richer after losses and tragedies than before his trouble.

As I worked through my experience, I have gained a real understanding of that message.

I have been blessed with a wonderful supportive family that has given me an immeasurable amount of love and has been a great source of pride to me. Support to my family from the community has given us a great source of strength. My misfortune has been insignificant and has added depth to my life's experiences. To have overcome a major threat to my health and accompanying disability gives me a deep sense of accomplishment. I know I could not have been successful without the help of the Lord. Just as the burning bush became a window for Moses to be aware of the presence of God, my illness and subsequent recovery have afforded me that same opportunity.

This experience has given my life more meaning. The Lord helps those who acknowledge Him and those who bring honor to Him by living according to His laws. I now understand how Job experienced a more bountiful life after his losses.

The human spirit is unique in its flexibility and resourcefulness. We all have the capacity to be what God wants us to be. It is important that we recognize that God is the director of the play and, as a result of his incomparable love for us, we are allowed to be the players.

The question is not "why me," but rather "why not me?" My illness presented me with a challenge. It was important that I meet it to serve as an effective role model to my children. However, my response was not one of choice. It was a result of the unwavering prayer support from my community and my family that gave me a sense of strength and confidence as I adjusted to the change in my life.

Henry Roberts and I reviewed my conclusion one evening by the fireside in our family room.

"Isn't the lesson of Job one of faith?" he asked.

"I can remember feeling the Lord's presence in my hospital room. Every time Mary Lynn came into my room I knew she had been sent to me as an inspiration, and meeting her and marrying her was not just a matter of luck."

"Don't you feel Job was more blessed because he knew God after his misfortunes?"

"You think I don't?"

Henry smiled and got up and hugged me.

In reviewing my experience, I have relived the frustrations and horror my wife endured. She went through a living hell! However, I believe there was a purpose to my failure to pursue discovery in a timely fashion. Had I sought damages or claimed disability, it would have been difficult to return to active practice. I would have been robbed of the immense satisfaction of overcoming a major disability. I enjoy my service to my patients and those who have known me longest say I am a better doctor because of my experience. They believe I am more sensitive and that patients relate to me better because they sense I have been on their side of the fence.

One of the most amazing features of the human experience is the ability to recover from a loss and bounce back from adversity. In order for function to be restored, one must go through a series of emotional responses that are well known to psychiatrists. Whether the loss is due to the death of a loved one or loss of function as in a disability due to illness or injury, one initially has a period of denial followed by depression. It is then essential to express grief or anger in order to recover from the depression. Then the healing process is enhanced by a period of rationalization. After the inner emotions are expressed, resignation or acceptance can occur.

Through the first six years, I went through some of these stages. Denial and depression were early stages. Then rationalization set in. I was driven by a terrific sense of thankfulness and resignation. I felt I had many things left to accomplish. There was no point in worrying about things I couldn't control. I was very thankful for the things I could do and for my loving family. I had accepted without question the reassurances I had received from the attending physicians, and my loyalty to Metropolitan Hospital was unshakable. However, after review of my chart, I can appreciate some of the emotions that divorced couples must feel. I am haunted by voices.

"It was a screwy case," as if it were my fault.

"You got first-class care."

"Don't you know how hard it is to diagnose renovascular hypertension?"

"There have to be nurses' notes somewhere!"

"Haven't you ever made a mistake?"

"You know I took the blood pressure."

They know I have questions and they know I've seen the chart. But one voice rings louder than the rest and puts everything in perspective: "Boy, you're lucky to be alive!" It is over. I don't judge them. I not only forgive them, I acknowledge there is nothing to forgive. It was a tough call and one that would have been missed by many of us. Cases like mine go with the territory. We all make mistakes.

I hope the lessons of my journey will help others recognize that we all must continually evaluate ourselves and recognize we are all human and subject to moments of weakness. We will not, and cannot, always be right, but we must aspire to that level of excellence.

If I had gone through the court system and been assigned damages and retired, I would never have had the opportunity to tell this story. I hope that patients everywhere will benefit from improved communications between health care professionals who all have the same goal — high-quality patient care and the commitment to improving that care.

It would have been very difficult for the jury to be sympathetic to my current handicaps. I am working full-time, I can ski, play golf and do almost anything I could do before my illness, although perhaps not quite so well.

I have taken my boys to our cabin in the North for fantastic fishing experiences. I am reminded of a verse that points out that, on a train trip through the rolling countryside, the destination or arrival at the station is not nearly so interesting or meaningful as the journey.

Life is an aggregate of experiences, just as a painting is a collage of color, a symphony a composition of notes and chords, and a novel, a portrayal of vignettes.

I am living my life to its logical end. Where the tracks lead is not clear. Any organization to life is imparted by the Director above, not by the players.

The players must try to keep their roles in the proper perspective. It is up to each of us to make sense of the conflicts in our lives. As we resolve our conflicts, we must understand that another observer may have a totally different interpretation of the meaning of the drama.

It is up to the observer to bring meaning to the production. Just as the observer makes the picture complete, it is up to each of us to bring understanding to our lives.

The importance of the observer was classically portrayed by Jan van Eyck, the Flemish master painter, in his portrait of Giovanni Arnolfini and his bride.

Close attention to the mirror, conspicuously placed behind the couple exchanging vows in the bridal chamber, reveals two witnesses. One of them is likely the painter himself, as the words above the mirror tell us Johannes de Eyck fuit hic (Jan van Eyck was there). The portrait by itself is only half the story. The other half is the audience.

Only the rules of the journey are distinct. We must follow

the tracks to their natural conclusion, limited only by how we treat our fellow passengers. With regard for our fellow man, our only constraint, we must be true to ourselves.

Many years ago, while in college, I was enjoying a weekend of golf with a fraternity brother, Morgan Metcalf, in El Dorado, Kansas. I had not played well and had been in trouble all day. My score had been respectable, but I spent most of the afternoon in the rough or other hazards, and I was continually having to invent a shot to get my ball back into the fairway. As we were sitting down to dinner with my friend's parents, his father, a physician, asked about our golf.

"Oh, I took the scenic route!" I replied.

Dr. Metcalf laughed out loud, "I'll have to remember that. That's the best description of a trying round of golf I've ever heard!"

THIRTY-ONE

VIETNAM VET TO JOIN COMRADES ON MEMORIAL

The headline caught my eye in the mid-1980s. I began reading as I do most articles about Vietnam since my one-year tour of duty as a battalion surgeon in 1968-69. As I read the story of Freddie Paul Heugel, I began to sense a re-awakening of a long suppressed memory. There was a hint of a memory of a wound I treated one night when our battalion had been the target of a Viet Cong mortar attack that came from a stronghold just over the Cambodian border, a few kilometers away.

It was a horrible wound. Most of the boy's left buttock had been shot away. As I lifted him onto the litter, I could feel the wound had penetrated his spinal cord.

The lead paragraph made me take a deep breath. "On Veteran's Day, more than 20 years after enemy mortar blew away most of his body below the waist, Freddie Paul Heugel will rejoin his comrades who sacrificed their lives in Vietnam."

"It couldn't be," I said to no one in particular.

"What did you say?" Mary Lynn was in the room.

I told her I was reading a story about a Vietnam casualty that sounded hauntingly familiar.

I read the article, which described the courage of a young man with a mortar wound to the left buttock, which resulted in an amputation of the left leg and eventually 8 percent of the spine with associated bowel and kidney damage.

The young man amazingly survived the surgery and went on to live a courageous life as an invalid. The story described his involvement in his community and total lack of bitterness toward the Army or his country that had agreed to disagree about the war in which he had fought.

"I think I was the first doctor that treated that soldier," I told Mary Lynn, "I don't know how to prove it. I left all my papers with the unit."

"Maybe I can help," Mary Lynn said. "I saved all your letters."

"The article says this boy was wounded on February 23, 1969," I told her.

She found a stack of letters all numbered. I smiled as I tried to promise myself to always watch what I wrote to her in the future. We struck pay dirt with a letter dated February 25, 1969. Excerpts from the letter confirmed my memory was not flawed.

"The situation remains much the same, although we've had no concentrated rocket or mortar attacks since I last wrote. I finally got to bed about 2300 on the 23rd, only to be wakened at 0300 to go to the hospital to meet a dust-off from Katum. The V.C. hit our radio bunker with two direct hits. One man was killed instantly and another was hit bad in the low back. I hauled them off the chopper here. The medics and I spent a long time cleaning the wounds up and maintaining an intravenous line for transfusions. I've never seen wounds as bad as these two had. Am afraid the injured one will be paralyzed from the waist down if he survives at all. He's in pretty bad shape. After he stabilizes, he'll be medivaced to Japan for neurosurgical care. Finally I got to bed again at 0600. It was a long three hours."

I reread the Livonia, Michigan newspaper article. It mentioned a Dr. Truman Strong, a dentist who had worked with Rep. William Ford of Michigan to cut through the red tape to allow Freddie's name to be added. I called Dr. Strong and asked him to relay to Mrs. Heugel that someone remembered and cared.

A few days later Mrs. Heugel called and told me the dedication ceremony would be on Veteran's Day at the Vietnam Memorial in Washington, D.C. "We are supposed to be there at 12:00. The ceremony is at 1:00. Can you be there?"

"I'll have to make some changes in my schedule," I told

her. I wasn't going to let a second lieutenant who had been four years old in 1969 represent Freddie's unit. "I'll do my best."

I thought of the battalion commander, Lt. Col. Robert W. Sennewald. I had heard he had made general and might be stationed near Washington. I knew he would be there if I could find him.

I called the V.F.W. and a friend of mine in the Medical Service Corp. at Fort Riley. The V.F.W. said they couldn't help on such short notice. My friend at Fort Riley, Col. Bill Speer, himself wounded in Vietnam, had his personnel officer work on finding Gen. Sennewald.

He called a few days later. "He's not on active duty. We're trying to run down a location on retired officers." I knew what I must do. I told Mary Lynn to pack for a weekend in Washington.

The night before we were to leave, Col. Speer called. "My personnel officer gets a gold star. He found someone who had a list of retired officers. The office in charge told him Sennewald was on the list, but he couldn't give any information because we didn't have a need to know.

"My man called back and told the secretary he hadn't written down General Sennewald's hometown. The secretary quickly said, 'Alexandria' before she realized what was going on. The rest was up to Ma Bell." He then gave me General Sennewald's phone number and address.

I called him the next morning and told him about SP/4 Freddie P. Heugel, assistant gunner, "C" Battery, 6/15 Artillery. He was moved that I planned to be there, after acknowledging he thought he remembered me out of a host of medical officers he had served with over the years. I told him I was to meet the family at noon at the memorial.

"I'll be there," he said. "I can't stay for the ceremony, but I'll see you at noon."

I knew someday I would go to the Wall. I thought of some names I might see. I would pay my respects to Sgt. John Thiery and Capt. Duncan McIntyre. Captain Mac was a battery commander I met the first week of my tour. He had an attitude of concern for his men that was reassuring. We talked of his interest in safety and attention to medical care. One visit was all I would have. Capt. Duncan McIntyre was killed a week later by an enemy mortar's direct hit in the very bunker we had visited.

In Washington, I was amazed at the number of people milling around. The attraction of the wall was magnetic. People were continually moving out of the crowd to peer closely at the inscribed names. The black facing provided a mirror-like effect, and the faces of the visitors and comrades were reflected back as a reminder of the adoration of the fallen soldiers.

The memorial seemed to embrace the crowd mixed with relatives and veterans with invisible arms. Many of the veterans were dressed in camouflage uniforms adorned with patches and unit logos. I realized it was going to be difficult to meet with Gen. Sennewald.

There were thousands of people moving around. Most were slowly moving by the wall looking for the names of their loved ones. There was a hostess in charge of a locator book to help find the location of a name of a loved one from a list of more than 58,000 names.

I had a clear vision of Lt. Col. Robert Sennewald in 1969. I tried to decide what Gen. Sennewald looked like in 1989. Would he be in uniform? I decided to stay in one spot. I wished we had been more particular about our reconnaissance.

I stood by the locator book. The hostess was pleasant company. I looked at the faces of all who filed by. They were a somber lot. All seemed to know where they were going. I decided to look for someone who looked as disorganized as I felt. Nobody seemed lost or confused. Finally I saw a Sgt. Major in uniform and asked if a retired general would wear a uniform to a ceremony such as this. "If it still fits him," he said quickly. The hostess guided me to a waiting area where some of the families gathered. Rep. Ford's secretary introduced herself and asked me to follow her to an area near the memorial that had been designated as reserved seating for the families of the veterans whose names were to be dedicated to the memorial at the ceremony.

She introduced me to Truman Strong, who took me over

to a gray-haired lady with a soft, pleasant smile. "This is Freddie's mother," he said in greeting. I put an arm around her in acknowledgment of our common sorrow "I know you had a long battle. I want you to know we were with Freddie immediately after he was hit. I wish we could have done more."

Words were not coming easily. It had been 20 years. As hard as I tried, I could not remember more than the wound. Mrs. Heugel had some pictures with her in a small album. There were pictures of Freddie in his specially equipped van, several pictures of him on his stomach on a hospital gurney, which he could propel with his arms.

"He lived on his stomach for 15 years," Dr. Strong said in explanation. Then Mrs. Heugel showed me a picture of Freddie in uniform, before he went to Vietnam. I was struck dumb. The picture of that boy, eyes fixed on the camera, opened up a closet in my mind I had closed and marked "off limits."

Tears started to fill my eyes. My voice failed me. I remembered a night 20 years ago. I remembered telling a young man how bad his wound was. I remembered he didn't seem to be frightened. He made my job easy. I only had to get the intravenous started for the blood transfusions. We had to dress the wound and apply pressure dressings and get his blood pressure up so he could be prepared for surgery. We did not have to spend much time comforting him. He was a tough kid.

"It's okay, doc. I'll be all right." He seemed to be more interested in reassuring me. I wished I could tell his mother what I felt. She looked at me as if she knew. I told her Gen. Sennewald was in the crowd. "He wanted me to tell you we all remember Freddie. There are so many people here, I doubt we'll make connections." Dr. Strong's wife wanted some pictures of me and Mrs. Heugel. I was overcome by the memories and emotions of the experience.

There was some activity on the speaker's platform. People were gesturing that families should be seated. The crowd began to fall into place behind the families. Once again, I told Mrs. Heugel I was sorry she hadn't met Gen. Sennewald.

A loud voice interrupted my train of thought. "Excuse me, I'm looking for the Heugel family." I turned and instead of a crowd of people, there was one man walking toward the designated seating area. I took two steps toward him. "Over here, sir."

The sir came out as a matter of habit. I caught my right arm as it responded as it had been programmed. Just as the salute began to crystallize, I caught it and offered my hand to Gen. Robert W. Sennewald. "Hello, doc, of course I remember you."

I turned to Mrs. Heugel. "Mrs. Heugel, I'd like to introduce you to Freddie's commanding officer. Then he was Lt. Col. Sennewald, now retired Gen. Sennewald." Gen. Sennewald put his arm around Mrs. Heugel. "I'm so sorry about your son," he said. "We don't have a good way of keeping track of our wounded. I understand he lived a very courageous life."

There were more pictures. Then Gen. Sennewald said, "I've decided to stay for the ceremony. I'll be back in the crowd. You stay with the family. I'll talk to you after the program."

The ceremony was fitting and solemn. There were remarks by Sen. Warner of Virginia and Jan Scruggs, a veteran of Vietnam who had been instrumental in the tribute to Vietnam veterans. The names of 19 additional veterans were read by a sister of one of the men, taps were played and it was over.

I had a strange feeling of fulfillment. The night of February 23, 1969, was the longest night of my life. It was finally over. I spoke with Mrs. Heugel again and thanked her for letting me share a special time with her.

Gen. Sennewald came up behind me. We talked a few minutes about old memories. He could not hide the tell-tale redness in his eyes, nor did he try. "The public does not suppose we feel," he said simply. "This is a special day."

"I believe I heard you were in line for promotion to general several years ago. I thought it best to introduce you as general rather than colonel. Was I right?" He looked back at me and nodded. "Four-star," was all he said.

We exchanged addresses and promised to stay in touch. I

believe we will. We have more to say to each other, but it was Freddie Paul Heugel's day. I took Mary Lynn by the hand and went to the locator book. I had one more thing to do.

The hostess was as pleasant as before. "The Mc's are after the M's," she said. I found the names. The hostess handed me a slip of paper with two penciled inscriptions: Section 27W – line 67 and section 37W - line 23. There were 72 lines on each section with 8 to 10 names per line. I quickly estimated that 6,000 soldiers had died during my tour of duty. Mary Lynn and I joined the throng at the wall. I paid my respects to two friends from 20 years before.

As I walked away from the Vietnam Memorial and looked at the Washington Monument and the Lincoln Memorial, I had an exhilarating feeling. Capt. Duncan B. McIntyre, Sgt. John Thiery and SP/4 Freddie Paul Heugel have come home. They are now recognized veterans who gave their lives for our country. The horrible wound is now diminished in my mind. Now, my most vivid memory of Vietnam is of a young man's courage, a mother's love, a general who cared and three names on a wall.

THIRTY-TWO

WHEN DRIVING in unfamiliar territory and with changing conditions, there are signs that serve to chart the course. We all have the potential to find the right direction if we heed the signals.

Spring mornings are made for sleeping. The windows were open and the breath of spring was in the air. Mary Lynn brought me coffee and the newspaper. "You're sleeping a little later this morning. I heard you get up in the night and knew you had gone to the emergency room."

I looked at the clock and saw it was 8:30. "I don't think I'll have time to get to church today. I have to make rounds, so I better get a move on." I showered quickly and had toast and cereal for breakfast. I made quick rounds at the hospital and went by the nursing home to see a few of my senior patients.

I checked the time and remembered church was at the Ottawa University Chapel as it was graduation weekend and the baccalaureate service was at the university. I decided it was too late for me to attend, but I remembered it was broadcast on the local radio, so I turned on the service when I got into the car. I had timed it perfectly as the sermon was beginning.

"You can't experience grace with a clenched fist," the minister began. A young girl in the prime of her life left her hometown in northern Michigan without even a good-bye. The small town was boring and she had fallen in with a fast crowd. She started smoking, using alcohol and did drugs. Finally she ran off to Detroit to get an apartment and really live. A missing persons report was filed by her parents with the local police. She didn't look back. Her parents grieved, but not a word. The authorities could not find a trace. The fast crowd in her hometown had some contacts in Detroit that provided shelter for her. Initially she was buoyed by the instant gratification of the chemical high, but soon she ran out of money. A part-time job only put her in contact with other desperate people. Finally her only choice was prostitution. She felt herself sinking. The despair was enveloping her."

I listened to the story intently as I drove into the driveway at home. As I stopped and reached for the key, I had a sense of comfort. Suddenly my life seemed to focus. The voice of the minister had seemed strangely familiar. I looked at the radio to be sure I had the local station, but I knew it was not our usual minister. Then it came back to me. I had heard that voice before; it was Roger Fredrickson, a graduate of Ottawa University, who had been the Baptist minister when I had been a youth. He was a member of the board of trustees at Ottawa University and was back to deliver the baccalaureate message.

"She felt her only hope was to try to swallow her pride and throw herself on the mercy of her father. She went to a pay phone and put a quarter in. It was late and no answer. She left a message, 'Daddy, I'm coming home. The bus stops at 1 a.m. tomorrow night. Meet me if you can; if you can't, I'll understand.'

"As she took the bus, she decided if her parents weren't there it meant they didn't want her back. She would stay on the bus and disappear into Canada. Then she wondered what if they were out of town or something had happened to them. When the bus stopped at her hometown bus station, she knew her prayers were answered. A huge banner was across the front of the depot, 'Welcome Home, Baby.' Tears ran down her cheeks she ran up to her father. She had her apology all ready. 'Daddy, I'm sorry, I ...' Her father's hand went over her lips, 'Sweetheart, there is not time for that, we have a lot of celebrating to do.' The story is a 1990s version of the Prodigal Son.

"I pause to congratulate the Class of 1998. It is with a lot of emotion that I address you today. My brother, Gerry, would have graduated with the Class of 1958, but he was killed in a car accident in his sophomore year. I spent some time lamenting that the driver and two others in the car walked away from the accident. There had been a question of alcohol. Last year my wife Ruth said to me, 'Roger, there is something you need to do.' I knew immediately what she meant. I picked up the phone and dialed information for a small Nebraska town and asked for the number of the driver of the van that Gerry was riding in. I dialed the number. A woman answered and told me her husband had died of Hodgkin's disease the year before. We must all learn to put conflict behind us and not to put off what needs to be done today."

Roger's message was clear. I had lived too long with a conflict in my life. I went in the back door and told Mary Lynn I was going into the den to take care of some old business. My letter began:

Dear Dr. Ford:

For some time I have planned to ask you to understand my poor communication as I struggled to put my life back together after my stroke. Being unable to drive limited my ability to address my concerns personally. I asked for and received my chart because of family comments that the nurses seemed confused and inattentive during my early hospitalization. When I saw a nearly 12-hour gap in nurses' notes, I felt it was an issue that surely must have been addressed. As I approach a time in my career that I want to wind down comfortably, I have come to realize that charting is haphazard at best.

A friend of mine met you several years ago at a Cystic Fibrosis fund raiser and told me you said you thought I blamed you for my illness. I want to settle that account. I was unfair to sound ungrateful. I was confused, as at that age I thought I was bulletproof. Having returned to practice and arrived at a point where I can comfortably retire in a year or so is a testimony to the care you provided 20 years ago. I am sorry for any discomfort I may have caused you.

Sincerely,
Bud Gollier

It was nearly a month later and after another trip to the

Northwest Territories that a letter from Dr. Ford arrived.

Dear Bud:

I am sorry to be late in returning your letter of May 24, but I spent a couple of weeks in Ireland in early June and am just getting settled back again. I found your letter to be moving in that it both saddens and in a way comforts me. I certainly appreciate your taking the time to write me. Over the years, I have looked back on your catastrophic illness, and in spite of the terrible things that it did to you, I can honestly say I felt your medical care, both in the Intensive Care and out of it, was very good. When you were in a hypertensive crisis, the care was exemplary. Again, I appreciate you writing to me in a very direct and honest manner. I am glad to hear you are going to be able to retire in a year or so and I am hoping to do so also. Very best personal regards, Bud.

Sincerely,
Chuck

Closure is fulfilling. As I read Dr. Ford's letter, I was sure Big Daddy, Dr. Delp and Dr. Drake all would have approved. Just as they had taught care of the patient and accountability, they held compassion, mercy, intellectual honesty and forgiveness as essential ingredients in the complete physician. The meaning of the scripture in the sixth chapter of Luke was clear. I have had the privilege of practicing medicine over 30 years. I will practice Christianity until I am called. The next Sunday, the scripture lesson spoke to me again. From the Gospel of Mark 4:21-24: 21:

And he said unto them. Is a candle brought to be put under a bushel or under a bed? and not to be set on a candlestick?

22 *For there is nothing hid, which shall not be manifested; neither was anything kept secret, but that it should come about.*

23 *If any man have ears to hear, let him hear.*

24 *And if he said unto them, Take heed what ye hear, with*

what measure ye mete, it shall be measured to you: and onto you that hear shall more be given.

A hearing ear and willingness to be led are essential for fulfilling God's plan.

THIRTY-THREE

Big NELLE is reluctant to talk about the changes in health care. She remembers an easier time and prefers not to discuss changes. "This too, will pass," she would say. But occasionally I challenge her to see if she will reflect on what my father may have done with the current system and how or whether he would deal with it. I stopped for coffee after church the Sunday before Christmas. "Mom, patients don't have choices anymore." She seemed relieved I wasn't there to tell her of the death or serious illness of one of her friends. "With managed care I have ceased to be a physician. I am now a gatekeeper. I open the gate to let the patient into the system if the patient meets the admission criteria. If they don't qualify for hospital admission or referral to a specialist, I treat them as I always have."

"Isn't that the way it has always been? Some people want to start with the specialist."

"What do you do if they ask you to send them on?"

"I try to tell them that I am a specialist, too, that I specialize in primary care and that I didn't make the rules."

"Can't they pay more and see the specialist anyway?"

"Certainly, some HMOs have an out-of-the-network coverage that will pay part of the fee, but it doesn't cost anything if I authorize the referral."

"Why don't you do it?"

"Because most illnesses do not require a specialist, and if I referred everyone, then the additional cost would break the system as it would cost much more than the politicians and insurance companies predicted."

"Sounds like your father."

"Dad would have hated it as much as I do. I spend half my time explaining the system to my patients. I have to explain co-pays, second opinions, the cost of pharmaceuticals, deductibles and what is covered and not covered when it comes to laboratory and outpatient services."

"Don't you pay someone to explain those things to your patients?"

"Sure, but they ask me first, and I'm better at it anyway, but it takes time away from patient care."

"Isn't that patient care?"

"Yes, I suppose it is, but it's not health care and it takes away from my primary responsibility."

"It sounds like the only thing that is different is that it takes more time."

"No, there are some other issues that worry me."

"Like what?"

"Patients have lost their individuality. Their diseases are not unique or personal. The diagnosis and plan of care must fit protocols. Every managed care plan issues its own set of practice protocols, which list suggested laboratory studies and treatment options for each disease.

"Do you have to follow these protocols?"

"Not yet. Now they are called guidelines. But make no mistake, they are going to be the standard covered service, and other plans of care will not be covered."

"It sounds awful."

"It may get worse. The managed care plans are already evaluating doctors by assessing their cost to the plan, and some plans are rewarding their most efficient doctors with bonuses for limiting costs. This provides an incentive for limiting services."

"What can patients do about it?"

"Take better care of themselves. One of these days it will occur to insurance companies to offer an incentive plan to promote regular physicals and smoking abstinence. The patients with the most devastating illnesses are those who have been uninsured or chosen to avoid check-ups with mammograms, Pap smears and cholesterol checks."

"Why do people do that?"

"Some people choose to avoid the system for a variety of personal reasons. Some religious, but most are economic. Some people are reluctant sheep. They are the challenges for the gatekeeper. They still want to choose, whether it be their doctor, their plan of care or whether to be treated at all."

"What can you do to encourage more people to participate?"

"I have had women refuse mammograms after I have recommended them and they come to the office with an obvious breast cancer. In one of those patients, the insurance company reviewed the chart and noted I had recommended the study, but felt I should have insisted the patient have the study done. I don't know how to do that. I asked the insurance company's medical director, a former practicing physician, why insurance companies didn't insist patients have a certain list of studies done each year to qualify for coverage." He said the companies would have to merge to define a risk pool to accomplish that. He had quit thinking like a doctor. He was now thinking like an administrator."

"Where's it going to end?"

"Probably with a lot of rules and regulations written by bureaucrats. With the huge national debt, the government is going to look at cost first. Everyone decries the cost of health care in the United States, and a figure of 14 percent of the gross domestic product is used with most of the Western European countries at 6 percent to 9 percent. Administrative costs are estimated at one-third of our health care costs. Add the 15 percent estimated for defensive medicine out of fear of malpractice, we have 50 percent of our cost unrelated to health care. That brings us in line with other civilized countries, and we have arguably the best health care in the world. What we must do is find a way to provide basic coverage for everyone, but we must keep regulators out of it. They will simply write more regulations to justify their own existence and drive those of us who try to take care of people crazy while they're at it."

"Your father would understand."

My youngest son will soon understand. John decided he wanted to be a doctor despite awareness of the stress in physicians' lives. He seemed undaunted by the long hours of study in his first year of medical school, and he didn't seem to have much free time.

Bo was comfortably progressing in his second year of dental school, and Sara Jane was in her senior year at K.U. making plans for a student teaching assignment in Kansas City. John was struggling with the question of primary care and specialization.

The spirit of Christmas filled the air. The minister set the tone at the Christmas Eve service at the First Baptist Church. Christmas Eve service was special to me. I had been baptized on Christmas Eve after I moved back to Ottawa. The children were baptized on Christmas Eve as well. The pastor spoke of the meaning of Christmas and gave thanks for redemption.

Before dinner on Christmas day, John came into the living room and sat down. I was reading the paper.

"Dad, I really like cardiology, but I don't want to live in a city. Don't you think the Clinton Health Plan will be a good deal for both doctors and patients? You'll be paid more if everyone has insurance and you won't have to worry about taking care of the uninsured patients for nothing."

"John, it will be a disaster. Reform is essential, but we can't expect to achieve a savings if the government controls it like they have Medicare."

"What do you mean?"

"Patients will lose the type of close care they have grown to expect, and they must have free choice of their physicians. If reform is to work, coverage must be universal and there must be no pre-existing illnesses that would limit coverage if an employee changes jobs."

"Won't the government have to fund the program?"

"Yes, but in order for reform to work, the patients must have some ownership of the health care system. There must be a basic premium for all through the insurance program, and co-pays must be a part of each encounter.

"If the government covers everyone without patient fiscal responsibility, doctors' offices will be overwhelmed, perhaps with phantom illnesses from people wanting a doctor's excuse from work or school.

"If the government covers everyone without patient responsibility, the administrative burden will eat up the savings and the employer mandates will be a disaster for small businesses. One coronary bypass operation will overwhelm an employer who doesn't have enough patients to enter a risk pool that allows for a major illness.

"Rural areas with fewer doctors will have problems as doctors won't have the time to share the administrative burden regarding chart review and utilization reports. Doctors have traditionally been involved in the administrative effort, but if doctors are overwhelmed seeing patients, they will not have the time to perform the administrative duty, and then the government will have to hire administrators to do the paperwork and these administrators will be paid high salaries and their costs will be charged to the cost of the entire program, and eventually doctors and hospitals will get the blame."

"Dad, I've been reading about the Oregon Plan, where health care is being rationed. Is that in the picture?"

"Eventually the choices will be to either limit reimbursement or ration health care. With regard to setting priorities and establishing a list of basic services, the legal profession will have a field day bringing lawsuits for discrimination against certain age groups or people with certain disabilities.

"That will be a very tough issue to address. And with the increase in administrative duties and the potential for limiting reimbursement, we will see fewer people choosing medicine as a profession, and the doctor shortage will become a major dilemma throughout the nation and not just in rural and inner city areas. We will find further deterioration of the doctor-patient relationship, and patients will have less say about the type of care they receive."

"What do you think about the Canadian single-payer system?"

"Canadians have made a number of serious mistakes. They elected to fund their program by taxation, and in Ontario the total tax rate for wealthy Canadians is close to 70% percent. There is now an entire generation of Canadians who have no idea of the cost or value of good health care.

"Many Canadian physicians are flooding to the United States because of the waiting list and the limitation of services they can perform. Their hospitals are struggling and having to cut services in a wholesale fashion. The Canadian system failed to address individual participation in the funding of the program."

John seemed uneasy, "What's wrong with the current system?"

"Premiums are too high. That's because of cost shifting and administrative costs. There are other factors that are important, but I feel those are the two major issues.

"Malpractice must be reformed. No one is denied care now. The main problem is that the cost of care limits access to care for many people. Too many people put off preventive care and early diagnosis because of the expense and lack of insurance. Then they end up in an emergency room or a hospital and that requires more expensive care, to say nothing of the loss of income during the time off the job."

"We have an excellent health care system with resources to provide the best care in the world. We simply must assure that it is available to everyone."

"What would you do?"

"I would hope Congress can guarantee care for everyone and fund care through a basic premium, which is adjustable annually and a significant co-pay with the incentive of reduced co-pay and premiums for those people who practice preventive medicine and have annual physicals for screening that meets the guidelines of the American Cancer Society and the American Heart Association.

"Also, we should have reduced costs for those people who don't smoke. These people should be issued a gold card as they don't cost as much as people who do not live a healthy lifestyle."

"How would you reform malpractice insurance?"

"I would let the patient decide what product he or she wants to buy. My patients trust me. They shouldn't have to pay higher fees to cover my malpractice insurance. They are the consumers. They should have a choice of their coverage. When they buy an appliance, they generally have a one-year factory warranty. They are then offered a service contract for up to sixty months. They can choose to purchase that if they want. Patients should have two fee schedules to choose from. In the basic plan they will be covered for damages much like homeowners. If they are not going to sue me, they shouldn't have to absorb my high insurance costs. An adjuster and consumer price indexes cover loss. In the case of malpractice claims I would offer an arbitration panel composed of attorneys, physicians and consumer rights activists. If they want protection under the present day tort system, they have a different schedule. It would cost more to play the lottery."

"Why won't that work?"

"There is a strong lobby of lawyers, administrators and insurance executives who don't want the system to change, and many of the congressmen are lawyers. So I would guess it is an uphill fight. And that means health care costs will continue to go up and the doctors will get the blame."

"What about places like Ottawa?"

"We'll be able to maintain the doctor-patient relationship longer than most areas because our patients are our friends and neighbors, but it gets tougher as there are fewer of us."

"And what if it comes to rationing care and increased paperwork?"

"I'm going fishing. The problem is that there are significant numbers of doctors in my generation who may choose early retirement. That will further compound the shortages and increase stress. However, most of us like what we do and want to continue the challenge of medicine, and we also want to do what we can to preserve that special commitment that doctors and patients share."

"What do you think makes doctors want to continue to work the long hours and subject themselves to the risks of malpractice?"

"I have thought about that a lot. Every time I'm on call, every phone call represents a potential $3-million-dollar suit. We have to do something about malpractice, but there are many benefits to the practice of medicine.

"The incentive to continue practicing in this environment is not related to the income. I don't make as much as a rag-armed minor league baseball pitcher. Satisfaction is a lot of it, but that's not all. Largely, it's a matter of conscience and doing a job well. I'll continue to practice as long as the system allows me to do my best. If mandates and protocols preempt my professional judgment, I'm gone."

"What did you mean when you said it's a matter of conscience?"

"Mahlon Delp always insisted that there were three rules to the practice of medicine — care of the patient, care of the patient and care of the patient. I think that he meant — care of the patient, care of the patient and care *for* the patient. I think we're obligated to provide the same sort of care for our patients that we would expect to receive ourselves.

"I think this commitment is a hard commitment for doctors to easily give up. It's a very special relationship, and it is developed through many years of committed physicians and a like involvement of the public. We must be careful to preserve the strengths of this system.

"Inside everyone's head is a little voice and when we do something that is contrary to the values we have learned, the little voice says, 'Don't do that.' And if we do it again, the little voice repeats the warning in a softer voice, and if we continue to compromise our values, the little voice stops talking to us. I think through the years of hard work and commitment we all learn what our duties are. It makes the long hours and the stress tolerable."

"And yet, you said you might quit and go fishing."

"I've been caring for patients for 30 years. I do not intend to spend the rest of my career explaining to patients why we have lost our opportunity to be participants in our lives. When we lose our free choice, we become objects, part of the bottom line. No, John, when you spend more time looking where you've been rather than where you're going, it will then be time to hang it up. With each new program, I have had to compromise the values learned from Dr. Delp, Dr. Drake, Big Daddy and many others. There comes a time when compromise is no longer an option."

Everyone was gathering in the dining room. Mary Lynn stepped into the room. "Bud, the turkey is ready for you."

A sense of thankfulness came over me as I was carving the turkey. Mary Lynn and Big Nelle put the food on the table.

We clasped hands as we stood around the table filled with the Lord's bounty. I led the prayer.

"Our Father in Heaven:
We thank you for this special day.
We revel in its meaning and its promise.
We thank you for the memories of those whose chairs
are vacant.
And for their dreams.
On this day, we particularly thank you for those
who will fulfill the dreams of Big Daddy,
Of PoPo and MoMo
And of Jani.
The dream of striving for excellence.
We thank you for the promise of youth.
For their enthusiasm and commitment.
Above all, we thank you for your Son.
And the gift of redemption.
And promises to keep.